D1714213

RESEARCH AND PERSPECTIVES IN ALZHEIMER'S DISEASE

Fondation Ipsen

B.T. Hyman   J.-F. Demonet
Y. Christen   (Eds.)

The Living Brain
and Alzheimer's Disease

With 49 Figures and 8 Tables

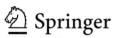 Springer

Hyman, Bradley T., M.D, Ph.D.
Neurology Service, Warren 408
Massachusetts General
Hospital/Harvard Medical School
Fruit Street
Boston, MA 02114
USA
E-mail: b-hyman@helix.mgh.harvard.edu

Christen, Yves, Ph.D.
Fondation IPSEN
Pour la Recherche Thérapeutique
24, rue Erlanger
75781 Paris Cedex 16
France
e-mail: yves.christen@beaufour-ipsen.com

Demonet, Jean-François, M.D.
Service Neurologie – Inserm U.455
CHU Hôpital Purpan
Place du Dr. Baylac
31059 Toulouse Cedex 3
France
E-mail: demonet@purpan.inserm.fr

ISSN 0945-6066
ISBN 3-540-21158-6 Springer-Verlag Berlin Heidelberg New York

Library of Congress-Cataloging-in-Publication-Data
The living brain and Alzheimer's disease / B.T. Hyman, J.-F. Demont, Y. Christen (eds.). p. ; cm.
(Research and perspectives in Alzheimer's disease) Proceedings of an intenational meeting, organized
by Fondation Ipsen, which took place in March 17, 2003. Includes bibliographical references and index.
   ISBN 3-540-21158-6 (alk. paper)
1. Alzheimer's disease – Diagnosis – Congresses.   2. Alzheimer's disease – Imaging – Congresses. 3. Brain
– Diseseases – Congresses.   4. Alzheimer's disease – Animal models – Congresses.   5. Brain – Animal mod-
els – Congresses.   6. Brain – Pathophysiology – Congresses.   7. Nervous system – Diseases – Diagnosis
– Congresses.   I. Hyman, B.T. II. Demont, J.-F. (Jean-Francois) III. Christen, Yves. IV. Series.
[DNLM: 1. Alzheimer Disease – diagnosis. 2. Alzheimer Disease – physiopathology. 3. Brain – physiopa-
thology. 4. Diagnosis Techniques, Neurological. WT 155 L 785 2004]

Springer-Verlag is a part of Springer Science+Business Media

springeronline.com

©Springer-Verlag Berlin Heidelberg 2004
Printed in Germany

The use of general descriptive names, registered names, trademarks, etc. in this publication does not imply,
even in the absence of a specific statement, that such names are exempt from the relevant protective laws and
regulations and therefore free for general use.

Product liability: The publishers cannot guarantee the accuracy of any information about dosage and application contained in this book. In every individual case the user must check such information by consulting
the relevant literature.

Production: PRO EDIT GmbH, 69126 Heidelberg, Germany
Cover design: design & production, 69121 Heidelberg, Germany
Printed on acid-free paper   27/3130Re – 5 4 3 2 1 0

Preface

Throughout the history of studies of Alzheimer's disease, there has been a dichotomy between the observations made by careful clinicians evaluating patients' symptoms, cognitive function, and progression, weighing diagnostic and research issues, and the neuropathologist on the other hand, who has the final say with regard to diagnosis, but has very little to say about what has happened to the brain prior to autopsy. From large cross-sectional studies of autopsy material, it seems as if a time course of disease, at least on average, can be mapped out: a pattern of hierarchical vulnerability for neuronal loss and neurofibrillary tangles beginning in medial temporal lobe structures like the entorhinal cortex and hippocampus, proceeding through association areas. Plaques follow their own temporal course, with widespread cortical deposits occurring even early in a disease process. The whole process may well take twenty years, the first half of which may be without overt symptoms.

How can we link the critical observations performed at autopsy with the events that occur over the previous twenty years of the illness? This is the problem posed to a group of our colleagues who are using state-of-the-art neural imaging methods in patients and in animal models to illuminate the natural history of the disease – in the living brain.

The Fondation Ipsen thus organized an international meeting on this topic in March 17, 2003, and the proceedings are contained herein. The editors wish to thank Mrs. Jacqueline Mervaillie for the organization of the meeting and Mary-Lynn Gage for the editing of the book.

May 2004

Bradley T. Hyman
Jean-François Demonet
Yves Christen

Contents

Contributors

Aguilnaldo, Gilbert
Departments of Radiology and Psychiatry, Mount Sinai School of Medicine,
New York, NY, USA

Alexander, Gene E.
Department of Psychology, Arizona Alzheimer's Disease Consortium,
1111 East Mc Dowell Road, Phoenix, AZ 85006, USA

Antoni, Gunnar
Uppsala University, PET Centre/Uppsala Research Imaging Solutions AB,
Uppsala , Sweden

Bacskai, Brian, J.
Massachusetts General Hospital, Department of Neurology/Alzheimer's Disease
Research Laboratory, 114 16th Street, No 2850, Charlestown, MA 02129, USA

Barlettta, Julien
Department of Organic Chemistry, Uppsala University, Uppsala, Sweden

Baron, Jean-Claude
University of Cambridge, Department of Neurology, Addenbrooke's Hospital,
Box 83, Cambridge CB2 2QQ, UK

Bergström, Mats
Uppsala University, PET Centre/Uppsala Research Imaging Solutions AB,
Uppsala , Sweden

Blomqvist, Gunnar
Uppsala University, PET Centre/Uppsala Research Imaging Solutions AB,
Uppsala, Sweden

Caselli, Richard J.
Department of Neurology, Mayo Clinic Scottsdale, and Arizona Alzheimer's
Disease Consortium, 1111 East McDowell Road, Phoenix, AZ 85006, USA

Chen, Kewei
Department of Mathematics, Arizona State University,
Good Samaritan Positron Emission Tomography Center,
1111 East McDowell Road, Phoenix, AZ 85006, USA

Chételat, Gaël.
INSERM E 218-University–Cyceron, 1400 Caen, France

De Zubicaray, Greig
Centre for Magnetic Resonance, University of Queensland, Brisbane, QLD 4072,
Australia

Debnath, Manik
Departments of Radiology and Psychiatry, University of Pittsburgh, Pittsburgh,
PA 15213, USA

Delatour, Benoît
Laboratoire NAMC CNRS UMR 8620, 91405 Orsay, France

Desgranges, B.
INSERM E 218-University–Cyceron, 1400 Caen, France

Dittmer, Stephanie S.
Laboratory of Neuro Imaging, Brain Mapping Division, Department of
Neurology, UCLA School of Medicine, 710 Westwood Plaza, Los Angeles,
CA 90095, USA

Doddrell, David M.
Centre for Magnetic Resonance, University of Queensland, Brisbane, QLD 4072,
Australia

Duff, Karen
Nathan S. Kline Institutes, New York University, Orangeburg, NY 10962, USA

Duyckaerts, Charles
Laboratoire de Neuropathologie Raymond Escourolle, Association Claude
Bernard, CHU Pitié-Salpêtrière, 75013 Paris, and INSERM U 106, France

Elliott, James, I.
Department of Molecular Biophysics and Biochemistry, Yale University,
New Haven, CT 06510, USA

Engler, Henry
Uppsala University, PET Centre/Uppsala Research Imaging Solutions AB,
Uppsala , Sweden

Estrada, Sergio
Uppsala University, PET Centre/Uppsala Research Imaging Solutions AB, Uppsala, Sweden

Eustache, F.
INSERM E 218-University–Cyceron, 1400 Caen, France

Fox, NickC.
National Hospital for Neurology and Neurosurgery, Queen Square, London WC1N 3BG, UK

Frosch, Matthew P.
Massachusetts General Hospital, Department of Neurology/Alzheimer's Disease Research Laboratory, 114 16th Street, No 2850, Charlestown, MA 02129, USA

Girardot, Nadège
Laboratoire de Neuropathologie Raymoand Escourolle, Association Claude Bernard, CHU Pitié-Salpêtrière, 75013 Paris, and INSERM U 106, France

Gretener, Danielle
Division of Psychiatry Research, University of Zurich, Lenggstr. 31, 8029 Zurich, Switzerland

Hauw, Jean-Jacques
Laboratoire de Neuropathologie Raymond Escourolle, Association Claude Bernard, CHU Pitié-Salpêtrière, 75013 Paris, and INSERM U 360, France

Hayashi, Kiralee M.
Laboratory of Neuro Imaging, Brain Mapping Division, Department of Neurology, UCLA School of Medicine, 710 Westwood Plaza, os Angeles, CA 90095, USA

Herman, David
Laboratory of Neuro Imaging, Brain Mapping Division, Department of Neurology, UCLA School of Medicine, 710 Westwood Plaza, Los Angeles, CA 90095, USA

Hickey, Gregory, A.
Massachusetts General Hospital, Department of Neurology/Alzheimer's Disease Research Laboratory, 114 16th Street, No 2850, Charlestown, MA 02129, USA

Hock, Christoph
Division of Psychiatry Research, University of Zurich, Lenggstr. 31, 8029 Zurich, Switzerland

Holt, Daniel
Departments of Radiology and Psychiatry, University of Pittsburgh, Pittsburgh,
PA 15213, USA

Hong, Michael S.
Laboratory of Neuro Imaging, Brain Mapping Division,
Department of Neurology, UCLA School of Medicine, 710 Westwood Plaza,
Los Angeles, CA 90095, USA

Huang, Guo-Feng
Departments of Radiology and Psychiatry, University of Pittsburgh, Pittsburgh,
PA 15213, USA

Hyman, Bradley, T.
Neurology Service, Warren 408,
Massachusetts General Hospital/Harvard Medical School, Fruit Street,
Boston, MA 02114, USA

Jack, Clifford R. Jr.
Department of Radiology, Mayo Clinic, 200 First Street SW, Rochester,
MN 55905, USA

Janke, Andrew L.
Centre for Magnetic Resonance, University of Queensland, Brisbane, QLD 4072,
Australia

Kajdasz, Stephen T.
Massachusetts General Hospital, Department of Neurology/Alzheimer's Disease
Research Laboratory, 114 16th Street, No 2850, Charlestown, MA 02129, USA

Kewei, Chen
Department of Mathematics, Arizona State University, Good Samaritan Positron
Emission Tomography Center and Arizona Alzheimer's Disease Consortium,
1111 East McDowell Road, Phoenix, AZ 85006, USA

Klunk, William E.
Departments of Radiology and Psychiatry, University of Pittsburgh, Pittsburgh,
PA 15213, USA

Långström, Bengt
Uppsala University, PET Centre/Uppsala Research Imaging Solutions AB,
and Department of Organic Chemistry, Uppsala University, Uppsala, Sweden

Langui, Dominique
Laboratoire de Neuropathologie Raymond Escourolle, Association Claude
Bernard, CHU Pitié-Salpêtrière, 75013 Paris, and INSERM U 106, France

Li, Yongsheng
Department of Neurology, New York University School of Medicine,
550 First Avenue, New York, NY 10016, USA

Maddalena, Alessia
Division of Psychiatry Research, University of Zurich, Lenggstr. 31, 8029 Zurich,
Switzerland

Mathis, Chester A.
Departments of Radiology and Psychiatry, University of Pittsburgh, Pittsburgh,
PA 15213, USA

McLellan, Megan E.
Massachusetts General Hospital, Department of Neurology/ Alzheimer's Disease
Research Laboratory, 114 16th Street, No 2850, Charlestown, MA 02129, USA

Nitsch, Roger. M.
Division of Psychiatry Research, University of Zurich, Lenggstr. 31, 8029 Zurich,
Switzerland

Nordberg, Agneta
Geriatric Department, Karolinska Institute, Huddinge University Hospital,
Stockholm, Sweden

Papassotiropoulos, Andreas
Division of Psychiatry Research, University of Zurich, Lenggstr. 31, 8029 Zurich,
Switzerland

Reiman, Eric M.
Good Samaritan PET Center, Arizona Alzheimer's Disease Consortium,
1111 East McDowell Road, Phoenix, AZ 85006, USA

Rose, Stephen E.
Centre for Magnetic Resonance, University of Queensland, Brisbane, QLD 4072,
Australia

Sadowski, Marcin
Department of Neurology, New York University School of Medicine,
550 First Avenue, New York, NY 10016, USA

Sandell, Johan
Uppsala University, PET Centre/Uppsala Research Imaging Solutions AB,
Uppsala , Sweden

Scahill, Rachael I.
National Hospital for Neurology and Neurosurgery, Queen Square,
London WC1N 3BG, UK

Scholtzova, Henrieta
Department of Neurology, New York University School of Medicine,
550 First Avenue, New York, NY 10016, USA

Schott, Jonathan M.
National Hospital for Neurology and Neurosurgery, Queen Square,
London WC1N 3BG, UK

Semple, James
Centre for Magnetic Resonance, University of Queensland, Brisbane,
QLD 4072, Australia

Sigurdsson, Einar, M.
Departments od Psychiatry and Pathology,
New York University School of Medicine, 550 First Avenue, New York,
NY 10016, USA

Skoch, Jesse
Massachusetts General Hospital, Department of Neurology/Alzheimer's Disease
Research Laboratory, 114 16th Street, No 2850, Charlestown, MA 02129, USA

Sowell, Elizabeth R.
Laboratory of Neuro Imaging, Brain Mapping Division,
Department of Neurology, UCLA School of Medicine, 710 Westwood Plaza,
Los Angeles, CA 90095, USA

Tang, Cheuk Ying
Departments of Radiology and Psychiatry, Mount Sinai School of Medicine,
New York, NY, USA

Thompson, Paul, M.
Reed Neurological Research Center,
Laboratory of Neuro Imaging, Department of Neurology,
UCLA School of Medicine, 710 Westwood Plaza, Los Angeles, CA 90095-1769,
USA

Toga, Arthur W.
Laboratory of Neuro Imaging, Brain Mapping Division,
Department of Neurology, UCLA School of Medicine, 710 Westwood Plaza,
Los Angeles, CA 90095, USA

Turnbull, Daniel H.
Departments of Pathology, Radiology, and Skirball Institute of Biomolecular
Medicine, New York University School of Medicine, 550 First Avenue, New York,
NY, 10016, USA

Wadghiri, Youssef Zaim
Skirball Institute of Biomolecular Medicine,
New York University School of Medicine, 550 First Avenue, New York,
NY 10016, USA

Wall, Anders
Uppsala University, PET Centre/Uppsala Research Imaging Solutions AB,
Uppsala , Sweden

Wang, Yanming
Departments of Radiology and Psychiatry, University of Pittsburgh, Pittsburgh,
PA 15213, USA

Wisniewski, Thomas
Departments of Psychiatry, Neurology and Pathology,
New York University School of Medicine, Milhauser Laboratory HN419,
550 First Avenue, New York, NY 10016, USA

Neuropathology of Alzheimer's Disease, as Seen in Fixed Tissues

Charles Duyckaerts[1,2], *Dominique Langui*[1,2], *Nadège Girardot*[1,2],
Jean-Jacques Hauw[1,3], *Benoît Delatour*[4]

Summary

The progress of in vivo imaging will in the future determine if deductions made from fixed tissue concerning the pathology of Alzheimer's disease (AD) were correct. It will mainly enable us to apprehend directly the chronological sequence of the lesions and their duration. This paper reviews some of the data concerning the classical pathology of AD. Lesions may be categorized into Aβ peptide deposition, tau accumulation and loss of neurons and of synapses. Aβ peptide originates from the amyloid precursor protein, a transmembrane protein that is found in lipid rafts of the cellular membrane. Accumulation of flotillin-1, a raft marker, in AD indicates a disturbance of this membrane transport system in AD. Diffuse deposits of Aβ peptide within the cerebral cortex have little clinical consequence. Focal deposits are generally amyloid, i.e., Congo red positive and highly insoluble. They are usually associated with microglial activation and low-grade inflammation. Aβ peptide is initially embedded in a cell membrane and partly hydrophobic. It may actually be linked to cholesterol in the extracellular milieu, as recently suggested. Tau accumulation takes place in the cell body, the dendrites and the axons of the neurons, forming, respectively, neurofibrillary tangles, neuropil threads and coronae of senile plaques. Heiko and Eva Braak have shown that the progression of neurofibrillary pathology takes place in a stereotyped manner that appears to be correlated with the clinical symptoms. Contrary to the prediction of the amyloid cascade hypothesis, neurofibrillary pathology in the rhinal cortex and pyramidal sectors of the hippocampus most often precedes the first morphological evidence of Aβ peptide accumulation. This observation suggests that tau and amyloid pathologies are, at the start, independent processes that secondarily interact. Data from transgenic mice support this view: neurofibrillary pathology is not observed in APP transgenic mice, except if a human mutated tau transgene has also been incorporated. Progression of the lesions is different in the entorhinal-hippocampal region and in the isocortex. In the former, tau pathology may be observed in the absence of Aβ deposition, which appears to be a relatively late phenomenon. In the isocortex, by contrast, Aβ peptide deposition is the first observable event.

---

[1] Laboratoire de Neuropathologie Raymond Escourolle, Association Claude Bernard, CHU Pitié,-Salpêtrière, Paris, France
[2] Inserm U 106
[3] Inserm U 360
[4] Laboratoire NAMC CNRS UMR 8620, Orsay, France

Hyman et al.
The Living Brain and Alzheimer's Disease
©Springer-Verlag Berlin Heidelberg

The sequence of the lesions in the isocortex appears to be the following: diffuse, focal, then amyloid deposits, neuropil threads, neuritic corona of the plaque and finally neurofibrillary tangles. Neuronal loss, in this sequence of events, occurs probably at a late stage, shortly preceding or occurring at the same time as tangle formation. Synaptic loss is a more complex process than previously thought: vesicular markers of the synapse drop sharply in advanced cases, whereas membrane markers are relatively spared. The decrease in the number of synapses is associated with enlargement of the ones that survive.

Up to now, observation of fixed brain tissue has dealt almost exclusively with proteins immobilized by formalin or other fixatives. Recent data show that membrane lipids play an essential role in the pathogenesis of AD. One of the future challenges of neuropathology will be to visualize not only the proteins but also the membrane domains that bear them.

Introduction

In 1902 and 1903, Max Bielschowsky described a new silver method that allowed him to visualize the "neurofibrils" (Bielschowsky 1902, 1903). Just a few years later, Alzheimer (Alzheimer 1907) and his pupil Perusini (1910) found what they

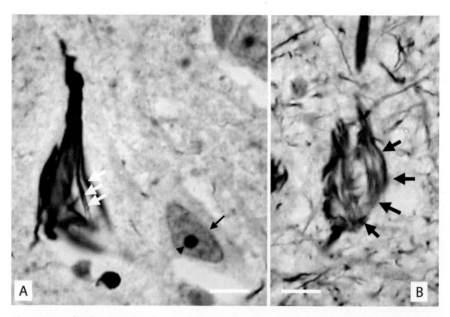

Fig. 1. Neurofibrillary tangles; **A** a neurofibrillary tangle, as stained by a silver impregnation (Bodian stain). The nucleus of a normal neuron (small arrow) and its nucleolus (arrowhead) is seen close to a tangle-bearing neuron. The tangle is indicated by large arrows. Bar = 10 μm; **B** a "ghost tangle," i.e., an extracellular neurofibrillary tangle (arrows). Ghost tangles are direct evidence of the death of tangle-bearing neurons.

initially thought was the pathology of the neurofibrils, i.e., the "neurofibrillary tangle." We know today that tangles are not made of neurofilaments, the protein that made the neurofibrils, but of tau protein.

Neurofibrillary Pathology

Neurofibrillary tangles kill the neurons (Fig. 1). A direct proof of this killing is the so-called ghost tangle, i.e., a tangle that is found outside the cell body of the neuron. Neurofibrillary tangles are quite common in the brain of aged people, but they are often confined to the entorhinal cortex and adjoining hippocampus (Fig. 2). They may constitute the only lesion visible in an aged brain. In many cases, according to the prevalence curves (Duyckaerts et al. 1997) drawn from Braak and Braak (1997) data concerning nearly 3,000 brains, the amyloid pathology follows tau accumulation in the neurofibrillary tangles. The mean delay between the two may be as long as 25 years (Duyckaerts et al. 1997).

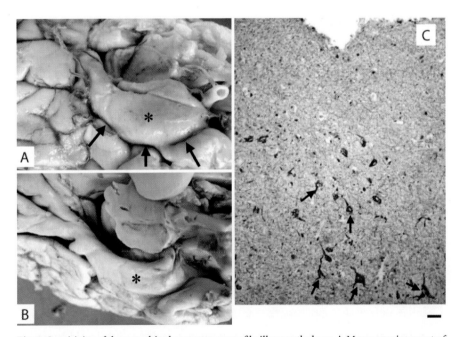

Fig. 2. Sensitivity of the entorhinal cortex to neurofibrillary pathology. **A** Macroscopic aspect of the entorhinal cortex in a normal case. The rhinal sulcus is shown by arrows. An asterisk indicates the external surface of the entorhinal area. **B** Atrophy of the entorhinal cortex. An asterisk indicates the surface of the entorhinal area. **C** Numerous ghost tangles (arrows) are seen in layer II of a case with atrophy of the entorhinal cortex. Bodian silver stain. Bar = 10 μm.

The Amyloid Pathology

The term amyloid has been used too extensively: in the strict sense, it means a Congo red- positive deposit that appears to be made of fibrils around 10 nm in diameter at electron microscopy (Fig. 3B, C). The Aβ peptide that precipitates in the cerebral parenchyma is initially not amyloid, and is shown only by immunohistochemistry (Fig. 3A). The peptide is the product of the cleavage of a large transmembrane precursor protein called amyloid precursor protein (APP). The first cleavage takes place in the exodomain and is due to the β-secretase activity attributed to the enzyme called BACE. The second cleavage occurs within the membrane domain and is related to an enzyme activity called gamma-secretase, linked to a multi-protein complex including presenilin 1, nicastrin, APH-1 and PEN-2 (Edbauer et al. 2003; Takasugi et al. 2003).

Aβ Peptide and APP

The cell(s) in which the Aβ peptide is produced, is (are) not fully identified. The neuron is, no doubt, involved, but the presence of Aβ peptide within the neuron has been documented only in a few instances in man (Chui et al. 2001), particu-

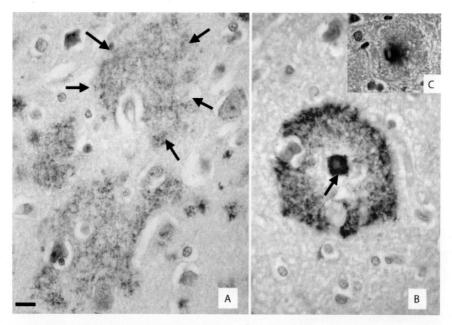

Fig. 3. Types of Aβ peptide deposits. **A** Diffuse deposits. One deposit is indicated by arrows. Immunohistochemistry of Aβ peptide. Avidin-Biotine-Peroxidase method. Chromogen : diaminobenzidine. Bar = 20 µm. **B** A focal deposit (arrow) is surrounded by a clear halo and an outer rim, less densely stained. **C** Congo red staining: the focal deposit shown in B is intensely congophilic.

larly in Down's syndrome (Gyure et al. 2001; Mori et al. 2002). Vesicles are also found in young transgenic APPxPS1 mice, before or at the time of the first deposits of Aβ peptide being seen (Wirths et al. 2001). These vesicles harbor markers of lysosomes and have their ultrastructural characteristics (Langui et al., manuscript in preparation). The stages of Aβ peptide production in the neuron are still incompletely known. APP, a transmembrane protein, has to be synthesized in the rough endoplasmic reticulum, the cellular organelle that allows the making of hydrophobic proteins or hydrophobic protein domains. The topography of Aβ production is still being discussed. It has been established that BACE acts before the gamma-secretase (Cupers et al. 2001; Maltese et al. 2001). It produces a fragment of APP (C99 or C100) that still contains the transmembrane domain and may then be subjected to gamma-secretase activity. This last cleavage takes place after the endoplasmic reticulum (Iwata et al. 2001; Maltese et al. 2001). Aβ peptide could then be liberated in the extracellular space by exocytosis or other mechanisms (Lam et al. 2001). It should be stressed, however, that a third of the length of the Aβ 42 peptide (namely its 14 last C terminal amino-acids) is probably still located in the membrane after the gamma-cleavage and is, anyway, hydrophobic. The presence of the pure peptide in the extracellular space is therefore improbable, and indeed a high content of cholesterol has been found in the core of the senile plaque (Mori et al. 2001; Girardot et al. 2003). The origin of the cholesterol in the plaque is still unknown. Apolipoprotein E, a transporter of cholesterol, is also present in the core of the senile plaque (Uchihara et al. 1995, 1996).

APP and the Lipid Rafts

APP is mobile in the cell membrane; it moves along the axon before being redistributed in the dendrites by transcytosis (Koo et al. 1990). The speed of its transport is not compatible with a passive diffusion. Cellular membrane is made of three types of lipids : glycerophospholipids, sphingolipids and cholesterol. At physiological temperature, the glycerophospholipids are above their melting point: they are "liquid,", actually in a "liquid crystalline" state. Sphingolipids, by contrast, are below their melting point in a "solid" state. Sphingolipids do not mix with glycerophospholipids. They form "microdomains" that are enriched in cholesterol. These "solid" microdomains float on the "liquid" glycerophospholipids of the membrane as rafts on water (for review see Fantini et al. 2002). Lipid rafts are of low density and sediment in the upper part of saccharose gradient. They are insoluble in Triton X-100 (Octyl phenol ethoxylate) at 4°C, a property that is used to isolate them. Five to 10% of neuronal APP are located at the cell membrane in lipid rafts (Bouillot et al. 1996). Recent data have suggested that the cytoplasmic domain of APP contains a kinesin receptor (Kamal et al. 2000, 2001). It links the raft to kinesin, which plays the role of a molecular engine mobile on the neurotubules. BACE (Riddell et al. 2001; Ehehalt et al. 2003) is also present in the raft fraction of the cell membrane. We have studied flotillin-1, a marker of rafts, in AD and found the accumulation of this marker in lysosomal vesicles of the neurons, a possible consequence of the disorganization of rafts (Girardot et al. 2003).

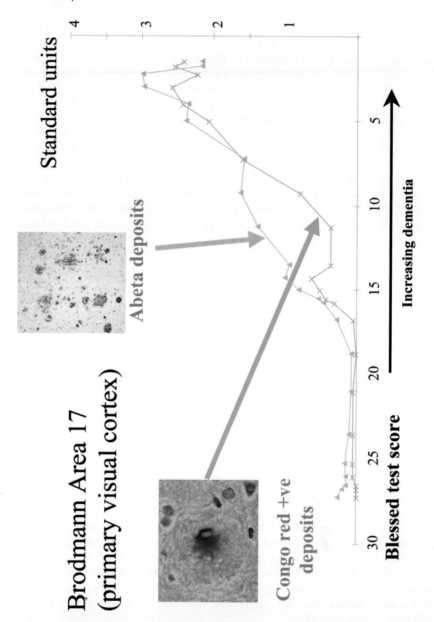

Fig. 4. Relationship between dementia and the density of Ab peptide deposits in Brodmann area 17. Intellectual status was evaluated in 26 cases (women aged over 75 years of age) by the test score of Blessed et al. (1968). Each point of the curve is a running mean of four successive cases (ranked in decreasing order of Blessed test score). The density of the Ab peptide deposits and of the Congo red-positive deposits, initially calculated as a proportion of volume, has been standardized [standardized value = (the original value - the minimal value over the whole co-hort)/standard deviation over the whole cohort]. Standardization allows comparison of values, which may differ by several degrees of magnitude. All the Ab deposits, whatever their shapes,

Diffuse and Amyloid Deposits

The distribution of Aβ peptide deposits in the isocortex is not as selective as the distribution of tau pathology. In most cases, Aβ deposits are, indeed, found in all the isocortical areas that are examined, an observation that suggests that the deposits occur almost simultaneously in the whole cerebral cortex. The deposits may be only diffuse without neuritic components. In those cases, the cognitive deficit is absent or minimal (Delaère et al. 1990; Dickson et al. 1991; Dickson 1997). In the study of a cohort of aged people, we used a cognitive index, the Blessed Test Score, as a time scale along which we plotted the density of the lesions (Metsaars et al. 2003). We showed that the presence of Congo red-positive plaques was detectable in cases that were only slightly more affected than those in which diffuse deposits of Aβ peptide were observed (Fig. 4). We could also show that the presence of Congo red-positive (amyloid) material was tightly associated with the presence of macrophages (Arends et al. 2000), that in turn initiate the inflammatory response. A receptor complex is involved in the detection of fibrillar Aβ by the microglial cell (Bamberger et al. 2003).

The Neuritic Plaque

Only at a more advanced stage is the central core of the amyloid plaque surrounded by a corona of degenerating neurites (Fig. 5); still later neurofibrillary tangles are detectable in the isocortex (Fig. 6). The neurites, which make up the corona of the senile plaque, could be axons or dendrites. Since they contain synaptic vesicles (Terry et al. 1964), are immunostained mainly by antibodies directed against phosphorylated neurofilaments (present in the axons), and are negative with antibodies against MAPs (present in dendrites; Schmidt et al. 1991), the conclusion has been drawn that they are mostly axonal terminals. However, the neurons from which these axons stemmed remained unclear, although indirect evidences pointed to the involvement of cortico-cortical connections (Duyckaerts et al. 1986).

The Innervation of the Neuritic Plaque

Transgenic mice gave us the opportunity to test this possibility in vivo. Biotinylated dextran amine (BDA; Brandt and Apkarian 1992; Veenman et al. 1992; Reiner et al. 1993) was used as an anterograde tracer to visualize axonal tracts and normal or dystrophic terminal boutons in transgenic mice with numerous Aβ peptide deposits. Ten aged (between 14 and 24 months) double transgenic mice, carrying the Swedish and London APP mutations and the PS1 M146L mutation (collaboration with Aventis Pharma), were used. The tracer was injected either in

---

were taken into account. Notice that the curve describing amyloid formation is close to the one describing Ab deposition. This observation suggests that amyloidogenesis occurs shortly after the accumulation of Ab peptide in the extracellular space.

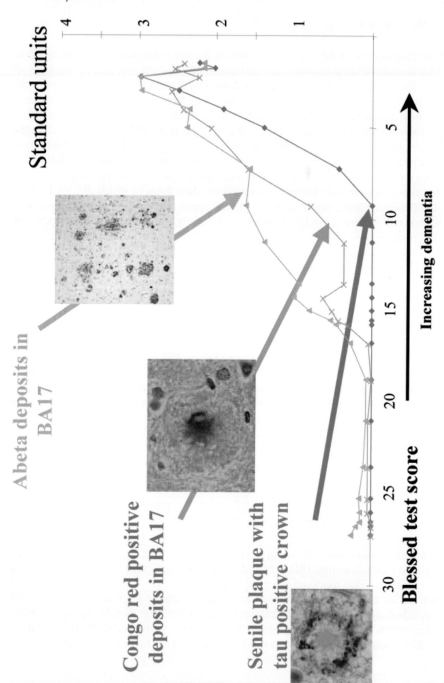

Fig. 5. Relationship between the Aβ peptide and the amyloid deposits and the corona of the senile plaque. Same methods as in Figure 4. Notice that the deposits surrounded by tau-positive processes occur at a later stage than the amyloid (Congo red-positive) deposits.

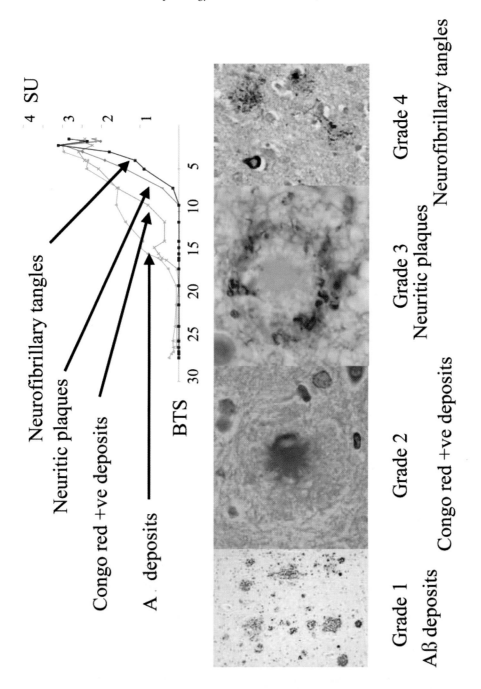

Fig. 6. Relationship between neuritic plaques and neurofibrillary tangles. Same methods as in Figure 4. The neurofibrillary tangles occur shortly after neuritic plaques, but there are samples with neuritic plaques without tangles.

the thalamus or in cortical areas (cingulate cortex, hippocampus). A high density of labeled neurites surrounding amyloid plaques was observed close to the injection site. These swollen, distended neurites were often observed in grape-like clusters around plaques. Not only short cortico-cortical axons (such as CA1-subicular connections) but also long-distance fiber association pathways (such as cingulo-frontal fibers that course the whole caudo-rostral extent of the brain to reach their targets) showed marked morphological alterations in relation to amyloid deposits. In other animals, the tracer was iontophoresed in subcortical areas (septal and thalamic nuclei). In all brains examined, only a very small number of degenerating neurites was observed at the level of cortical axonal terminal fields. For example, despite very dense projections from the mediodorsal thalamic nucleus to the plaque-enriched prefrontal pole, no clear evidence of pathological boutons was seen close to the amyloid deposits in this cortical area. We concluded that the senile plaques were mainly innervated by cortico-cortical connections (Delatour et al. 2003).

Pathological Grades

As there is a sequence in the order of involvement of the cortical areas, there is a sequence of lesions affecting a given isocortical area: diffuse deposits of Aβ peptide precede amyloid formation, neuritic plaques and finally neurofibrillary tangles. This sequence can be used to grade the lesions within a given area (Metsaars et al. 2003; Fig. 7).

Synaptic and Neuronal Loss

Synaptic loss has been considered the best correlate of dementia (Terry et al. 1991), although this has been questioned (Dickson et al. 1995). The vesicular markers of the synapse, such as synaptophysin, are much more severely affected than the membrane markers (Shimohama et al. 1997).

Neuronal loss is often considered a major correlate of dementia. Its evaluation is difficult and subjected to numerous methodological problems. No neuronal loss could be observed when the total number of neurons was evaluated in the cerebral cortex (Regeur et al. 1994). On the contrary, neuronal loss was found to be severe when the analysis was restricted to well-circumscribed areas, such as layer II of the entorhinal cortex or the cortex bordering the superior temporal sulcus (Gomez-Isla et al. 1996, 1997). We tried to evaluate the laminar topography of the neuronal loss by using a method that assesses the area around each neuron rather than the number of neurons per area. When the neighbors of a neuron are far apart, the free area around it is large and the cellular density is low (Duyckaerts et al. 1994, 2000). The measure of the free space surrounding each neuron is a local measurement of the density. The "numerical density of one neuron" is the ratio 1/(the area left free around that neuron). This area is the region of space that is closer to that neuron than to any other. It has the shape of a polygon, called a Voronoi (or Dirichlet) polygon, the sides of which are located at mid-distance from

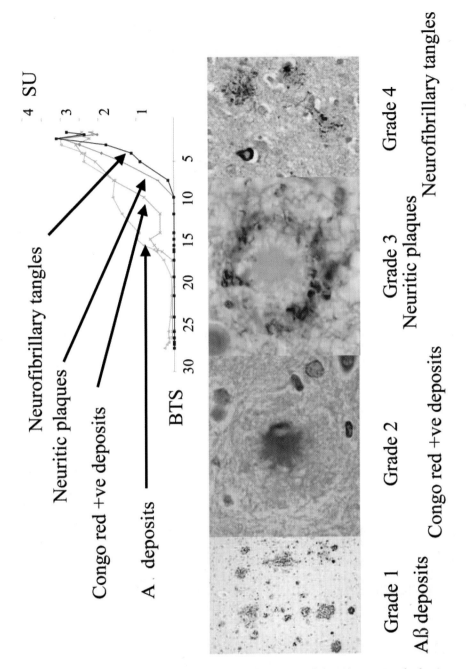

Fig. 7. The four grades of the lesions as proposed by Metsaars et al. (2003). SU = Standard unit. The grading system, applicable only in the isocortex, is based on the detection of characteristic lesions, the progression of which is indicated by the curves.

the neighboring cells. The Voronoi polygons are contiguous and their set fills the space without interstice or overlap - i.e., they perform a "tessellation." Using Voronoi tessellation, we showed that the neuronal loss in the cerebral cortex mainly involved the supragranular layers (occupied by neurons involved in cortico-cortical connections). The interindividual variability of neuronal density is, however, high a finding that renders difficult the assessment of its chronological sequence. In our cohort of cases, we could not precisely determine when the neuronal loss appeared. However, we were able to show that the borderline that maximized the difference in neuronal density between the cases was at a neurofibrillary tangle density of 5 neurons / mm2 (Grignon et al. 1998).

Conclusions

A neuropathologist, examining a slide of fixed tissue, has many reasons to feel frustrated. His vision is indeed limited, both in time and space. The picture that he gains from reality is obtained through a complex and fragile chain of deductions. We have presented here data that might enable him to imagine the progression of AD in the brain from the observation of fixed tissue: the neurofibrillary tangles in the hippocampus and entorhinal cortex precede the diffuse deposits of Aβ peptide in the isocortex. Some of these deposits become amyloid and these Congo red-positive deposits trigger an inflammatory reaction. Neuritic plaques and neurofibrillary tangles then appear in the isocortex and significant numbers of neurons are lost.

Will these observations be confirmed by in vivo imaging? Will in vivo imaging enable us to apprehend such important questions as: how much time does it takes for a tangle or a plaque to appear. How long do they stay in the brain? In which sequence and at what pace do they progress? The success of in vivo imaging will also be crucial to understand the diagnostic significance of the neurofibrillary tangles that are so common in aging. Can their number remain stable? Do they inexorably increase in number? Much of this information will obviously be necessary to devise new treatments.

Acknowledgments

Dominique Langui is presently financed by Réseau Alzheimer, Aventis Pharma®, which also supported Benoît Delatour. The help of Laurent Pradier and Véronique Blanchard (Aventis Pharma®) is greatly acknowledged. Nadège Girardot is the recipient of a grant from France Alzheimer.

References

Alzheimer A (1907) Uber eine eigenartige Erkrankung der Hirnrinde. Allgemeine Zeitschr Psychiatr Gerichtlisch Med 64: 146–148

Arends M, Duyckaerts C, Rozemuller JM, Eikelenboom P, Hauw J-J (2000) Microglia, amyloid and dementia in Alzheimer disease. A correlative study. Neurobiol Aging 21: 39–47

Bamberger ME, Harris ME, McDonald DR, Husemann J, Landreth GE (2003) A cell surface receptor complex for fibrillar beta-amyloid mediates microglial activation. J Neurosci 23: 2665–2674

Bielschowsky M (1902) Die Silberimprägnation der Achsencylinder. Neurologisches Zentralblatt (Leipzig) 21: 579–584

Bielschowsky M (1903) Die Silberimprägnation der Achsencylinder. Neurologisches Zentralblatt (Leipzig) 22: 997–1006

Blessed G, Tomlinson BE, Roth,M (1968) The association between quantitative measures of dementia and of senile change in the cerebral grey matter of elderly subjects. Brit J Psychiat 114: 797–811

Bouillot C, Prochiantz A, Rougon G, Allinquant B (1996) Axonal amyloid precursor protein expressed by neurons in vitro is present in a membrane fraction with caveolae-like properties. J Biol Chem 271: 7640–7644

Braak H, Braak E (1997) Frequency of stages of Alzheimer-related lesions in different age categories. Neurobiol Aging 18: 351–357

Brandt HM, Apkarian AV (1992) Biotin-dextran: a sensitive anterograde tracer for neuroanatomic studies in rat and monkey. J Neurosci Meth 45: 35–40

Chui DH, Dobo E, Makifuchi T, Akiyama H, Kawakatsu S, Petit A, Checler F, Araki W, Takahashi K, Tabira T (2001) Apoptotic neurons in Alzheimer's disease frequently show intracellularAbeta42 labeling. J Alzheimer's Dis 3: 231–239

Cupers P, Bentahir M, Craessaerts K, Orlans I, Vanderstichele H, Saftig P, De Strooper B, Annaert W (2001) The discrepancy between presenilin subcellular localization and gamma-secretase processing of amyloid precursor protein. J Cell Biol 154: 731–740

Delaère P, Duyckaerts C, Masters C, Piette F, Hauw JJ (1990) Large amounts of neocortical ßA4 deposits without Alzheimer changes in a nondemented case. Neurosci Lett 116: 87–93

Delatour B, Blanchard V, Pradier L, Duyckaerts C (2003) The innervation of senile plaques: a link between amyloid and neurofibrillary pathology? Annual on Alzheimer's disease and related disorders. London, Martin Dunitz, in press.

Dickson D (1997) Qualitative differences between senile plaques (SP) in pathological aging (PA) and Alzheimer disease. Brain Pathol 7: 1054

Dickson DW, Crystal HA, Mattiace LA, Masur DM, Blau AD, Davies P, Yen S, Aronson MK (1991) Identification of normal and pathological aging in prospectively studied nondemented elderly humans. Neurobiol Aging 13: 179–189

Dickson DW, Crystal HA, Bevona C, Honer W, Vincent I, Davies P (1995) Correlations of synaptic and pathological markers with cognition of the elderly. Neurobiol Aging 16: 285–304

Duyckaerts C, Godefroy G (2000) Voronoi tessellation to study the numerical density and the spatial distribution of neurones. J Chem Neuroanat 20: 83–92

Duyckaerts C, Hauw JJ, Bastenaire F, Piette F, Poulain C, Rainsard V, Javoy-Agid F, Berthaux P (1986) Laminar distribution of neocortical plaques in senile dementia of the Alzheimer's type. Acta Neuropathol (Berl) 70: 249–256

Duyckaerts C, Godefroy G (1994) Evaluation of neuronal numerical density by Dirichlet tessellation. J Neurosci Meth 51: 47–69

Duyckaerts C, Colle MA, Bennecib M, Grignon Y, Uchihara T, Hauw JJ (1997) Plaques and tangles: where and when? In: Hyman BT, Duyckaerts C, Christen Y (eds) Connections, cognition, and Alzheimer's disease. Berlin, Springer-Verlag, pp. 33–39

Edbauer D, Winkler E, Regula JT, Pesold B, Steiner H, Haass C (2003) Reconstitution of gamma-secretase activity. Nature Cell Biol, 5:486–488

Ehehalt R, Keller, Haass C, Thiele C, Simons K (2003) Amyloidogenic processing of the Alzheimer beta-amyloid precursor protein depends on lipid rafts. J Cell Biol 160: 113–123

Fantini J, Garmy N, Mafhoud R, Yahi N (2002) Lipid rafts: structure, function and role in HIV, Alzheimer's and prion diseases. Expert Rev Mol Med. www.expertreviews.org/02005392h. htm

Girardot N, Allinquant B, Langui D, El Hachimi KH, Dubois B, Hauw JJ, Duyckaerts C (2003) Accumulation of flotillin-1 in tangle-bearing neurones of Alzheimer's disease. J Neuropathol Appl Neurobiol. 29: 451-461

Gomez-Isla T, Price JL, McKeel DW, Morris JC, Growdon JH, Hyman BT (1996) Profound loss of layer II entorhinal cortex neurons occurs in very mild Alzheimer's disease. J Neurosci 16: 4491-4500

Gomez-Isla T, Hollister R, West H, Mui S, Growdon JH, Petersen RC, Parisi JE, Hyman BT (1997) Neuronal loss correlates with but exceeds neurofibrillary tangles in Alzheimer's disease. Ann Neurol 41: 17-24

Grignon Y, Duyckaerts C, Bennecib M, Hauw JJ (1998) Cytoarchitectonic alterations in the supramarginal gyrus of late onset Alzheimer's disease. Acta Neuropathol (Berl) 95: 395-406

Gyure KA, Durham R, Stewart WF, Smialek JE, Troncoso JC (2001). Intraneuronal abeta-amyloid precedes development of amyloid plaques in Down syndrome. Arch Pathol Lab Med 125: 489-492

Iwata H, Tomita T, Maruyama K, Iwatsubo T (2001) Subcellular compartment and molecular subdomain of beta-amyloid precursor protein relevant to the Abeta 42-promoting effects of Alzheimer mutant presenilin 2. J Biol Chem 276: 21678-21685

Kamal A, Stokin GB, Yang Z, Xia CH, Goldstein LS (2000) Axonal transport of amyloid precursor protein is mediated by direct binding to the kinesin light chain subunit of kinesin-I. Neuron 28: 449-459

Kamal A, Almenar-Queralt A, LeBlanc JF, Roberts EA, Goldstein LS (2001) Kinesin-mediated axonal transport of a membrane compartment containing beta-secretase and presenilin-1 requires APP. Nature 414: 643-648

Koo EH, Sisodia SS, Archer DR, Martin LJ, Weidemann A, Beyreuther K, Fischer P, Masters CL, Price DL (1990) Precursor of amyloid protein in Alzheimer disease undergoes fast anterograde axonal transport. Proc Natl Acad Sci USA 87: 1561-1565

Lam FC, Liu R, Lu P, Shapiro AB, Renoir JM, Sharom FJ, Reiner PB (2001) beta-Amyloid efflux mediated by p-glycoprotein. J Neurochem 76: 1121-1128

Maltese WA, Wilson S, Tan Y, Suomensaari S, Sinha S, Barbour R, McConlogue L (2001) Retention of the Alzheimer's amyloid precursor fragment C99 in the endoplasmic reticulum prevents formation of amyloid beta-peptide. J Biol Chem 276: 20267-20279

Metsaars WP, Hauw JJ, van Welsem ME, Duyckaerts C (2003) Pathology of tangle-free areas. A grading system of Alzheimer lesions in the isocortex. Neurobiol Aging 24: 565-574

Mori C, Spooner ET, Wisniewski KE, Wisniewski TM, Yamaguchi H, Saido TC, Tolan DR, Selkoe DJ, Lemere CA (2002) Intraneuronal Abeta42 accumulation in Down syndrome brain. Amyloid 9: 88-102

Mori T, Paris D, Town T, Rojiani AM, Sparks DL, Delledonne A, Crawford F, Abdullah LI, Humphrey JA, Dickson DW, Mullan MJ (2001) Cholesterol accumulates in senile plaques of Alzheimer disease patients and in transgenic APP(SW) mice. J Neuropathol Exp Neurol 60: 778-785

Perusini G (1910) Über klinisch und histologisch eigenartige psychische Erkrangungen des späteren Lebensalters. Histologische und histopathologische Arbeiten. Nissl F, Alzheimer A, Jena Gustav Fischer

Regeur L, Badsberg Jensen G, Pakkenberg H, Evans SM, Pakkenberg B (1994) No global neocortical nerve cell loss in brains from patients with senile dementia of Alzheimer's type. Neurobiol Aging 15: 347-352

Reiner A, Veenman CL, Honig MG (1993) Anterograde tracing using biotinylated dextran amine. Neuroscience protocols. Wouterlood, F. G. Amsterdam, Elsevier

Riddell DR, Christie G, Hussain I, Dingwall C (2001) Compartmentalization of beta-secretase (Asp2) into low-buoyant density, noncaveolar lipid rafts. Curr Biol 11: 1288-1293

Schmidt M, Lee V, Trojanowski J (1991) Comparative epitope analysis of neuronal cytoskeletal proteins in Alzheimer's disease senile plaque, neurites and neuropil threads. Lab Invest 64: 352–357

Shimohama S, Kamiya S, Taniguchi T, Akagawa K, Kimura J (1997) Differential involvement of synaptic vesicle and presynaptic plasma membrane proteins in Alzheimer's's disease. Biochem Biophys Res Commun 236: 239–242

Takasugi N, Tomita T, Hayashi I, Tsuruoka M, Niimura M, Takahashi Y, Thinakaran G, Iwatsubo T. (2003) The role of presenilin cofactors in the gamma-secretase complex. Nature 422: 438–441

Terry RD, Gonatas JK, Weiss M (1964) Ultrastructural studies in Alzheimer presenile dementia. Am J Pathol 44: 269–297

Terry RD, Masliah E, Salmon DP, Butters N, DeTeresa R, Hill R, Hansen, LA, Katzman R (1991) Physical basis of cognitive alterations in Alzheimer's disease : synapse loss is the major correlate of cognitive impairment. Ann Neurol 30: 572–580

Uchihara T, Duyckaerts C, He Y, Kobayashi K, Seilhean D, Amouyel P, Hauw JJ (1995) ApoE immunoreactivity and microglial cells in Alzheimer's disease brain. Neurosci Lett 195: 5–8

Uchihara T, Duyckaerts C, Lazarini F, Mokhtari K, Seilhean D, Amouyel P, Hauw JJ (1996) Inconstant apolipoprotein E (ApoE)-like immunoreactivity in amyloid beta protein deposits: Relationship with APOE genotype in aging brain and Alzheimer's disease. Acta Neuropathol (Berl) 92: 180–185

Veenman CL, Reiner A, Honig MG (1992) Biotinylated dextran amine as an anterograde tracer for single- and double-labeling studies. J Neurosci Methods 41: 239–54

Wirths O, Multhaup G, Czech C, Blanchard V, Moussaoui S, Tremp G, Pradier L, Beyreuther K, Bayer TA (2001) Intraneuronal Abeta accumulation precedes plaque formation in beta- amyloid precursor protein and presenilin-1 double-transgenic mice. Neurosci Lett 306: 116–20

Cerebrospinal Fluid Biomarkers for the Diagnosis of Alzheimer's Disease

Andreas Papassotiropoulos[1], Alessia Maddalena, Danielle Gretener,
Roger M. Nitsch, Christoph Hock[1]

Summary

The antemortem diagnosis of probable Alzheimer's disease (AD) requires time-consuming and costly procedures. Therefore, biomarkers that can direct the physician rapidly to the correct diagnosis are highly desirable. According to the consensus report of the working group on "Molecular and Biochemical Markers of Alzheimer's Disease," the ideal biomarker for AD should have a sensitivity of >80% for detecting AD and a specificity of >80% for distinguishing other dementias. Candidate diagnostic markers were identified by quantitating proteins associated with the characteristic histopathological hallmarks of AD: β-amyloid plaques and neurofibrillary tangles (NFT). Cerebrospinal fluid (CSF) levels of amyloid β-peptide (Aβ42) and total tau protein, as well as combinations of the two, were shown to corroborate the clinical diagnosis of AD; however, they did so without fully meeting the working group guidelines. Combined CSF measurements of phosphorylated tau protein (phospho-tau) and Aβ42 and calculation of the phospho-tau/Aβ42 ratio resulted in a further, slight improvement of diagnostic accuracy (Maddalena et al. 2003). Thus, measurement of the CSF phospho-tau/Aβ42 ratio meets the working group guidelines for sensitivity and comes close to meeting the guidelines for specificity. It is currently unclear how both sensitivity and specificity values can be set at levels higher than 90%. It is unlikely that this goal can be achieved by measurement of Aβ peptides and tau proteins alone, because the AD neuropathology is characterized by a variety of other lesions, such as infarcts, gliosis, argyrophilic grains and Lewy bodies. Moreover, the neuropathology of other dementing conditions, such as frontotemporal lobe dementias, displays partially AD histopathological features.

Among numerous biomarkers proposed so far, only those associated with the characteristic histopathological hallmarks of AD – b-amyloid plaques and neurofibrillary tangles (NFT) - have been shown to be valid and to corroborate the clinical diagnosis of AD. In the cerebrospinal fluid (CSF), the levels of the amyloid b-peptide 1–42 (Aβ42) are found to be low in AD patients, whereas the CSF levels of the microtubule-associated protein tau are high. The development of assays detecting hyperphosphorylated or pathologically phosphorylated forms of tau (phospho-tau) increased diagnostic specificity without, however, improving sensitivity. Recently developed proteomic technologies may ultimately lead to the

---

[1] Division of Psychiatry Research, University of Zurich, Lengstr. 31, 8029 Zurich, Switzerland

discovery of other CSF proteins that may complement the diagnostic repertoire and may be used for monitoring disease progression and therapeutic efficacy.

Cerebrospinal Fluid Aβ42

Motter et al. (1995) presented the first evidence of a decrease in Aβ42 levels in the CSF of AD patients. The reason for this decrease is not clear. Possible mechanisms may include the enhanced aggregation of Aβ42 in the brain, resulting in reduced solubility of this peptide in the CSF. Several subsequent studies replicated the initial results of Motter et al. However, although significantly different, low CSF Aβ42 levels in AD patents are of limited diagnostic utility, particularly due to an overlap with CSF Aβ42 values from cognitively healthy elderly and from patients with non-AD dementias. CSF levels of the shorter species Aβ40 failed to discriminate AD from normal aging or other dementias (Kanai et al. 1998; Mehta et al. 2000). In our study cohort of 100 outpatients that underwent diagnostic work-up for dementia in our memory disorders unit, we also observed that CSF Aβ42 levels are significantly lower in AD patients as compared to cognitively healthy control subjects, patients with non-AD dementias and patients with other neurological disorders (Maddalena et al. 2003; Table 1).

In contrast to CSF, plasma levels of Aβ42 were reported to be elevated in AD, particularly in carriers of presenilin mutations (Scheuner et al. 1996). However, further studies demonstrated that elevated plasma levels of Aβ42 do not reliably differentiate between AD, other dementias and normal aging, due to considerable overlap between the groups (Mehta et al. 2000; Table 2).

Cerebrospinal Fluid Total Tau

The microtubule-associated protein tau is abundant in the human central nervous system (CNS) and is expressed predominantly in axons, where it binds to and stabilizes microtubules (MTs; Lee et al. 2001). Tau is physiologically phosphorylated at many sites, including those flanking the MT binding regions, and it is well established that increasing tau phosphorylation negatively regulates MT binding (Biernat et al. 1993; Bramblett et al. 1993; Drechsel et al. 1992). In the human brain, regions affected early in AD (e.g., hippocampus) show significant tau pathology (Braak and Braak 1991). Several studies have reported an increase of tau levels in the CSF of AD patients, possibly mirroring the degeneration of NFT-containing neurons (Arai et al. 1995; Hock et al. 1995; Kapaki et al. 2003; Vandermeeren et al. 1993). The elevation of CSF tau occurs early in AD and is stable over time, with low interindividual variation (Andreasen et al. 1999). However, due to a high degree of overlap between AD and other dementias, particularly tauopathies and Creutzfeldt-Jakob disease, the diagnostic usefulness of CSF tau as a single biomarker is limited (Table 3).

Table 1. CSF levels of Aβ42 (ng/ml)

Reference	AD patients	Healthy control subjects	Non-AD dementias	Other neurological diseases
Hulstaert et al. 1999	0.49 (0.39–0.62)[a]	1.00 (0.80–1.21)	0.60 (0.43–0.74)	0.77 (0.61–0.91)
Kapaki et al. 2003	0.36 (0.31–0.45)	0.74 (0.51–0.86)	0.52 (0.44–0.79)	–
Maddalena et al. 2003	0.42 ± 0.19	0.73 ± 0.22	0.64 ± 0.33	0.85 ± 0.33
Sjogren et al. 2000	0.38 ± 0.12	0.77 ± 0.24	0.49 ± 0.17	0.61 ± 0.17

[a] Values are given as mean ± standard deviation or median with upper and lower quartiles (in parentheses).

Table 2. Plasma Levels of Aβ42 (pg/ml)

Reference	AD patients	Healthy control subjects	Non-AD dementias	Other neurological diseases
Mehta et al. 2000	73 (25–880)[a]	81 (25–905)	–	–
Vandersticherle et al. 2000	121 ± 56	144 ± 104	127 ± 25	111 ± 17

[a] Values are given as mean ± standard deviation or median with upper and lower quartiles (in parentheses).

Table 3. CSF Levels of total tau (pg/ml)

Reference	AD patients	Healthy control subjects	Non-AD dementias	Other neurological diseases	MCI
Andreasen et al. 1999[a]	690 ± 341	227 ± 101	–	–	–
Buerger et al. 2002[a]	721 ± 352	247 ± 137	–	–	578 ± 258
Hulstart et al 1999[b]	425 (274–713)	219 (134–318)	220 (122–426)	160 (125–217)	[d]
Itoh et al. 2001[a]	858 ± 480	[e]	441 ± 260[f]	339 ± 181	–
Kapaki et al 2003[b]	504 (348–854)	140 (110–223)	173 (139–372)	–	–
Schonknecht et al. 2009[c]	578 (180–1200)	254 (80385)	273 (157–505)	–	–

[a] Values are given as mean ± standard deviation.

[b] Values are given as Medians with upper and lower quartiles.

[c] Value given as median with range.

[d] This study included four subjects with MCI. Due to this low number, mean values are not shown in the table.

[e] This study did not report detailed values for the group of healthy controls. According to the figures, the CSF levels of total tau in healthy subjects were comparable with the levels of the group with other neurogical diseases.

[f] Patients with frontotemporal lobe dementia.

Cerebrospinal Fluid Phospho-Tau

Hyperphosphorylation is possibly an early event in the pathway that leads from soluble to filamentous tau protein, finally resulting in the formation of paired helical filaments (PHF). In the AD brain, several protein kinases and phosphatases are implicated in the dysregulation of tau phosphorylation. In an attempt to increase the discrimination between AD and other dementias, refined assays were developed with antibodies specifically recognizing pathologically phosphorylated tau epitopes. The most widely used phospho-tau immunoassays recognize tau protein phosphorylated at threonine 181 (p-tau181; Vanmechelen et al. 2000), serine 199 (p-tau199; Itoh et al. 2001) and threonine 231 (p-tau231; Buerger et al. 2002). These assays have proven more specific than total tau assays and discriminate better between AD and diseases of the CNS that are also accompanied by total tau elevation in the CSF (e.g., Creutzfeldt-Jakob disease, meningoencephalitis and stroke). Moreover, CSF phospho-tau is found to be elevated in subjects with mild cognitive impairment (MCI), who are at increased risk to develop AD (Buerger et al. 2002). Despite this improvement, phospho-tau assays also fail to reach sensitivity and specificity values high enough to allow their routine diagnostic use (Table 4). By considering both sources of information (i.e., CSF Aβ42 and tau), some studies demonstrated improved diagnostic accuracy compared with CSF Aβ42 and CSF tau alone (Hulstaert et al. 1999; Kapaki et al. 2003; Maddalena et al. 2003). The measurement of the CSF phospho-tau/Aβ42 ratio comes close to the criteria of the working group on "Molecular and Biochemical Markers of Alzheimer's Disease" (National Institute on Aging 1997).

Conclusion

The discovery of new diagnostic tools based upon biochemical markers for AD is of major clinical importance. CSF levels of Aβ42 and tau protein, which are associated with the characteristic histopathological hallmarks of AD, were shown to corroborate the clinical diagnosis of AD, although not fully meeting the working group guidelines. It is currently unclear how both sensitivity and specificity values can be set at levels higher than 90%. It is unlikely that this goal can be achieved by measurement of Aβ peptides and tau proteins alone, because the AD neuropathology is characterized by a variety of other legions, such as infarcts, gliosis, argyrophilic grains and Lewy bodies. Morevover, the neuropathology of other dementing conditions, such as frontotemporal lobe dementias, displays partially AD histopathological features. The use of advanced proteomic technologies may lead to discovery of additional proteins of diagnostic relevance that may allow for setting up a diagnostic tool suitable for routine clinical use.

Table 4. CSF levels of phospho-tau (pg/ml)

Reference	AD patients	Healthy control subjects	Non-AD dementias	Other neurological diseases	MCI
Buerger et al. 2002	710 ± 373[a]	78 ± 114	–	–	501 ± 400
Itoh et al. 2001	150 ± 71	[b]	87 ± 47[c]	47 ± 32	–
Maddalena et al. 2003	52 ± 19	27 ± 10	37 ± 18	36 ± 15	–
Schonknecht et al. 2003	73 (41–172)	52 (28–69)	54 (31–83)	–	–

[a] Values are given as mean ± standard deviation or median with range (in parentheses).

[b] This Study did not report detailed values for the group of healthy controls. According to the figures, the CSF levels of phospho-tau in healthy subjects were comparable with the levels of the group with other neurological diseases.

[c] Patients with frontotemporal lobe dementia

Acknowledgments

This study was funded in part by the National Centre of Competence in Research on Neural Plasticity and Repair, the EU DIADEM programme on Diagnosis of Dementia, and the University of Zurich.

References

Andreasen N, Minthon L, Clarberg A, Davidsson P, Gottfries J, Vanmechelen E, Vanderstichele H, Winblad B, Blennow K (1999) Sensitivity, specificity, and stability of CSF-tau in AD in a community-based patient sample. Neurology 53: 1488–1494

Arai H, Terajima M, Miura M, Higuchi S, Muramatsu T, Machida N, Seiki H, Takase S, Clark CM, Lee VM, Trojanowski JQ, Sasaki H (1995) Tau in cerebrospinal fluid: a potential diagnostic marker in Alzheimer's disease. Ann Neurol 38: 649–652

Biernat J, Gustke N, Drewes G, Mandelkow EM, Mandelkow E (1993) Phosphorylation of Ser262 strongly reduces binding of tau to microtubules: istinction between PHF-like immunoreactivity and microtubule binding. Neuron 11: 153–163

Braak H, Braak E (1991) Neuropathological stageing of Alzheimer-related changes. Acta Neuropathol 82: 239–259

Bramblett GT, Goedert M, Jakes R, Merrick SE, Trojanowski JQ, Lee VM (1993) Abnormal tau phosphorylation at Ser396 in Alzheimer's disease recapitulates development and contributes to reduced microtubule binding. Neuron 10: 1089–1099

Buerger K, Teipel SJ, Zinkowski R, Blennow K, Arai H, Engel R, Hofmann-Kiefer K, McCulloch C, Ptok U, Heun R, Andreasen N, DeBernardis J, Kerkman D, Moeller H, Davies P, Hampel H (2002) CSF tau protein phosphorylated at threonine 231 correlates with cognitive decline in MCI subjects. Neurology 59: 627–629

Drechsel DN, Hyman AA, Cobb MH, Kirschner MW (1992) Modulation of the dynamic instability of tubulin assembly by the microtubule-associated protein tau. Mol Biol Cell 3: 1141-1154

Hock C, Golombowski S, Naser W, Muller-Spahn F (1995) Increased levels of tau protein in cerebrospinal fluid of patients with Alzheimer's disease--correlation with degree of cognitive impairment. Ann Neurol 37: 414–415

Hulstaert F, Blennow K, Ivanoiu A, Schoonderwaldt HC, Riemenschneider M, De Deyn PP, Bancher C, Cras P, Wiltfang J, Mehta PD, Iqbal K, Pottel H, Vanmechelen E, Vanderstichele H (1999) Improved discrimination of AD patients using beta-amyloid(1-42) and tau levels in CSF. Neurology 52: 1555–1562

Itoh N, Arai H, Urakami K, Ishiguro K, Ohno H, Hampel H, Buerger K, Wiltfang J, Otto M, Kretzschmar H, Moeller HJ, Imagawa M, Kohno H, Nakashima K, Kuzuhara S, Sasaki H, Imahori K (2001) Large-scale, multicenter study of cerebrospinal fluid tau protein phosphorylated at serine 199 for the antemortem diagnosis of Alzheimer's disease. Ann Neurol 50: 150–156

Kanai M, Matsubara E, Isoe K, Urakami K, Nakashima K, Arai H, Sasaki H, Abe K, Iwatsubo T, Kosaka T, Watanabe M, Tomidokoro Y, Shizuka M, Mizushima K, Nakamura T, Igeta Y, Ikeda Y, Amari M, Kawarabayashi T, Ishiguro K, Harigaya Y, Wakabayashi K, Okamoto K, Hirai S, Shoji M (1998) Longitudinal study of cerebrospinal fluid levels of tau, A beta1-40, and A beta1-42(43) in Alzheimer's disease: a study in Japan. Ann Neurol 44: 17–26

Kapaki E, Paraskevas GP, Zalonis I, Zournas C (2003). CSF tau protein and beta-amyloid (1-42) in Alzheimer's disease diagnosis: discrimination from normal ageing and other dementias in the Greek population. Eur J Neurol 10: 119–128

Klatka LA, Schiffer RB, Powers JM, Kazee AM (1996) Incorrect diagnosis of Alzheimer's disease. A clinicopathologic study. Arch Neurol 53: 35–42

Lee VM, Goedert M, Trojanowski JQ (2001) Neurodegenerative tauopathies. Annu Rev Neurosci 24: 1121–1159

Maddalena A. Papassotiropoulos A, Müller-Tillmanns B, Jung HH, Hegi T, Nitsch RM, Hock C (2003) Biochemical diagnosis of Alzheimer's disease by measurement of the cerebrospinal fluid phospho-tau/Aβ42 ratio. Arch Neurol 60:1195–1196

McKhann G, Drachman D, Folstein M, Katzman R, Price D, Stadlan EM (1984) Clinical diagnosis of Alzheimer's disease: report of the NINCDS-ADRDA Work Group under the auspices of Department of Health and Human Services Task Force on Alzheimer's Disease. Neurology 34: 939–944

Mehta PD, Pirttila T, Mehta SP, Sersen EA, Aisen PS, Wisniewski H M. (2000) Plasma and cerebrospinal fluid levels of amyloid beta proteins 1-40 and 1-42 in Alzheimer disease. Arch Neurol 57: 100–105

Motter R, Vigo-Pelfrey C, Kholodenko D, Barbour R, Johnson-Wood K, Galasko D, Chang L, Miller B, Clark C, Green R, Olson D, Southwick P, Wolfert R, Munroe B, Lieberburg I, Seubert P, Schenk D (1995) Reduction of beta-amyloid peptide42 in the cerebrospinal fluid of patients with Alzheimer's disease. Ann Neurol 38: 643–648

National Institute on Aging (1997) Consensus recommendations for the postmortem diagnosis of Alzheimer's disease. The National Institute on Aging and Reagan Institute Working Group on Diagnostic Criteria for the Neuropathological Assessment of Alzheimer's Disease. Neurobiol Aging 18: S1–2

Scheuner D, Eckman C, Jensen M. Song X, Citron M, Suzuki N, Bird TD, Hardy J, Hutton M, Kukull W, Larson E, Levy-Lahad E, Viitanen M, Peskind E, Poorkaj P, Schellenberg G, Tanzi R, Wasco W, Lannfelt L, Selkoe D, Younkin S (1996) Secreted amyloid beta-protein similar to that in the senile plaques of Alzheimer's disease is increased in vivo by the presenilin 1 and 2 and APP mutations linked to familial Alzheimer's disease. Nature Med 2: 864–870

Schonknecht P, Pantel J, Hunt A, Volkmann M, Buerger K, Hampel H, Schroder J (2003) Levels of total tau and tau protein phosphorylated at threonine 181 in patients with incipient and manifest Alzheimer's disease. Neurosci Lett 339: 172–174

Sjogren M, Minthon L, Davidsson P, Granerus AK, Clarberg A, Vanderstichele H, Vanmechelen E, Wallin A, Blennow K2000) CSF levels of tau, beta-amyloid(1-42) and GAP-43 in frontotemporal dementia, other types of dementia and normal aging. J Neural Transm 107: 563–579

Vandermeeren M, Mercken M, Vanmechelen E, Six J, van de Voorde A, Martin JJ, Cras P (1993) Detection of tau proteins in normal and Alzheimer's disease cerebrospinal fluid with a sensitive sandwich enzyme-linked immunosorbent assay. J Neurochem 61: 1828–1834

Vanderstichele H, Van Kerschaver E, Hesse C, Davidsson P, Buyse MA, Andreasen N, Minthon L, Wallin A, Blennow K, Vanmechelen E (2000) Standardization of measurement of beta-amyloid(1-42) in cerebrospinal fluid and plasma. Amyloid 7: 245–258

Vanmechelen E, Vanderstichele H, Davidsson P, Van Kerschaver E, Van Der Perre B, Sjogren M. Andreasen N, Blennow K. (2000) Quantification of tau phosphorylated at threonine 181 in human cerebrospinal fluid: a sandwich ELISA with a synthetic phosphopeptide for standardization. Neurosci Lett 285: 49–52

The Living Brain and Alzheimer's Disease

Bradley T. Hyman[1]

The Diagnosis of Alzheimer's Disease

For nearly a century the definitive diagnosis of Alzheimer's disease has been based upon histopathological changes that can be observed only at autopsy. The marked neuronal loss and development of amyloid-containing extracellular plaques and Tau-containing intracellular neurofibrillary tangles have provided clues to the biology of Alzheimer's disease as well as insight into clinical-pathological correlations (Duyckaerts et al. 1998). However, we believe that it is now critical to move from histopathological diagnosis to diagnosis in the "living brain."

Why can't we do this already? Currently, the diagnostic criteria for Alzheimer's disease in living patients involve the clinical symptoms of dementia and "ruling out" other possible causes of cognitive decline. Clinicians in specialized centers can be "right" about the diagnosis of Alzheimer's disease about 9 times in 10. Current advances in biomarkers measured in the cerebrospinal fluid (CSF) may solidify or enhance these numbers (Hock et al. 1998). The problem, however, lies in two important issues.

The first has to do with the clinical decision-making involved in making a diagnosis of Alzheimer's disease. Since the clinical diagnosis is based on the presence of symptoms of memory loss, aphasia, apraxia, etc., these symptoms must be noticed by the patients or their family, they must be sufficiently severe to come to medical attention, and they must also be severe enough to seem "worse" than what is expected with normal aging. These are each difficult to define and vary enormously from population to population and even from doctor to doctor. Especially in the very first stages of the illness, when the symptoms are mild, quantitation of the degree of change becomes extremely challenging unless extensive longitudinal studies are performed. Even then, subtle changes from baseline on cognitive testing can reflect a variety of test-retest issues, as well as the impact of systemic disease, depression, or concurrent neurological diseases such as small strokes. As we look forward to an era in which we will have more and more effective anti-Alzheimer agents, it is becoming increasingly clear that measuring their efficacy with measures (such as performance on cognitive testing) that are sensitive to whether or not the patient has concurrent illnesses at best confounds analyses, and at worst can completely impair analysis. Quantitative neuroimaging

---

[1] Department of Neurology, Massachusetts General Hospital/Havard Medical School, Boston, Masachusetts

may prove to be a critical asset in therapeutic trial design (Alexander et al. 2002; Jack et al. 2003).

The second reason, however, is even more important. Our understanding of the natural history of Alzheimer's disease has progressed substantially in the last decade. It is now believed that the pathophysiologic process of Alzheimer's disease - that is, the deposition of amyloid plaques, the development of neuro-fibrillary tangles, and the loss of specific subpopulations of projection neurons - occurs long before clinical symptoms become overt. Most of this work is based upon cross-sectional autopsy studies, showing that the same pattern of alterations that occurs in Alzheimer's disease also occurs in non-demented elderly, but to a lesser extent in the non-demented elderly. Intensive analysis of individuals who happened to die while they were in the mildest cognitive impairment stages of Alzheimer's disease fits this pattern exactly: they have the same topographical pattern of neuropathology as seen in non-demented elderly or in Alzheimer's disease patients, but quantitatively fit right in the middle (Gomez-Isla et al. 1996). By making assumptions about the rate of accumulation of tangles or plaques, or the rate of loss of neurons in various brain areas, it has been estimated that the "disease process" occurs about a decade before even the mildest cognitive symptoms can be detected. Neuroimaging studies suggest detectable atrophy more than three years before symptoms (Schott et al. 2003).

Finally, because we do not yet have the ability to reverse neuronal damage that has already occurred, identifying Alzheimer's disease in the living brain will be critical to identifying, diagnosing, and intervening in individuals who have the brain changes of initial Alzheimer's disease, even before dementia occurs. As therapeutics are developed, the logic of going towards preventive strategies in individuals that are considered to be "presymptomatic" will be compelling. Only by identifying these biochemical and neuropathological changes *in the living brain* will we succeed.

Thus, these are the challenges we face: to detect in the living brain the lesions that, until now, have only been detected by histopathological analysis; to detect them early in the disease process, before clinical symptoms start; and to detect them quantitatively, so that the amount or rate of change of the lesions can be used to guide the development of therapeutics, and to guide their use.

The Neuropathological Changes of Alzheimer's Disease

Alzheimer described the presence of neurofibrillary tangles, senile plaques, gliosis, and neuronal loss in his initial case study. These four remain the primary histopathological features of Alzheimer's disease, although in recent years specific molecular identification of the lesions, and a better understanding of their topographic mapping throughout the brain, has been achieved. From the point of view of the "living brain," however, the changes can be divided into two broad categories: the "positive changes," in which something new appears, like amyloid deposits or neurofibrillary tangles, and the "negative changes," in which something that had been present disappears, like neurons or synapses. Because the positive changes lead to the appearance of new phenomena, they are attractive targets for imaging studies. In principle, the image would go from blank to having something on it. On the other hand, studies of atrophy (the sum of neuronal loss and synaptic loss) have appeal because of the extraordinary success of high resolution structural imaging, giving the ability to quantitate even quite subtle changes in the size or shape of brain regions, like the entorhinal cortex and hippocampus, or of broader cortical regions. Quantitative histopathological studies, especially those using stereology (Gomez-Isla et al. 1997), have defined brain regions at particular risk for atrophy early in the disease process and have led the way towards successful imaging protocols (Jack et al. 1998; Killiany et al. 2000). Thus, the histopathology guides us toward living brain imaging.

Studies on the Living Brain

Unlike histopathological studies that can only determine structure, studies of the living brain include assays of brain function. Because Alzheimer's disease is a disease that affects neural systems and is characterized by a breakdown in interactions between association areas and limbic areas, it has been believed that assessments of the functional integrity of these specific brain areas, perhaps while performing memory-related tasks, might amplify any structural changes that are present (Sperling et al. 2002).

Indeed, these strategies have proven extremely promising. Single photon emission tomography, positron emission tomography, regional cerebral blood flow, and functional MRI studies all reveal characteristic patterns of dysfunction in patients with Alzheimer's disease (Fazekas et al. 1989; Jagust et al. 1991; Sihver et al. 2000; Bradley et al. 2002). In recent years, multiple studies have demonstrated that some of these same patterns can be elicited earlier and earlier in the disease process. It seems likely that further advances in specific paradigms, as well as technological advances to enhance both quantitation and resolution of these images, will lead to an ability to monitor the "negative" aspects of Alzheimer's pathophysiology: loss of neurons, loss of synapses, and loss of functional neural system integrity.

Similarly, extraordinary advances in structural imaging and the ability to reconstruct images into three-dimensional sets, followed by a comparison of one brain to another or one brain to itself at a later time point, have led to the clear recognition that specific patterns of atrophy occur in Alzheimer's disease and even occur much earlier than clinical symptoms (Fox et al. 2001). The themes here are similar: development of new generations of technologies to increase the resolution of the scans and, perhaps even more importantly, development of newer technologies to compare one scan to the next so that subtle changes can be reliably followed (Thompson et al. 2001; Jack et al. 2003).

Until very recently, progress has been frustratingly slow in the development of imaging approaches for the positive lesions of Alzheimer's disease. Although neurofibrillary tangles and amyloid deposits likely populate the cortex a decade before symptoms occur, and are essentially absent in young brains, the ability to detect these lesions has been elusive. The reasons for this are two-fold: first, the lesions are truly microscopic (less than 100 micometers) and therefore well below the level of resolution of clinical imaging techniques; and second, the development of ligands that specifically bind to plaques or tangles and can cross the blood-brain barrier has been a difficult process. Part of the excitement in the field is the sense that we are on the threshold of overcoming these problems. Both PET ligands (Klunk et al. 2001; Klunk et al. 2002) and MRI contrast agents (Poduslo et al. 2002) are nearing the point where clinical use can be foreseen.

Based on histological dyes that are known specifically to bind amyloid plaques or neurofibrillary tangles, a new generation of PET ligands has emerged that has the promise of distinguishing Alzheimer patients from controls and of providing a quantitative estimate of the amount of amyloid in any brain region. This series of breakthroughs has also enabled other imaging modalities, including those specifically utilizing small animal models for Alzheimer's disease, to monitor amyloid deposition in the living brain in these model systems (Christie et al. 2001). This technique provides an outstanding platform to test new therapeutic approaches, especially to try to "reverse" the amyloid deposits (Bacskai et al. 2001). It seems likely that further development of the ligands will lead not only to PET tracers but also to contrast agents that may be applicable for more widely available imaging technologies such as SPECT or MRI.

What we can Learn

Why is so much effort going into trying to find ways to image Alzheimer disease pathology, when the diagnosis can be made with an accuracy of 9 out of 10 by an experienced clinician? The critical issue is to develop technologies that will enable us to not simply diagnose Alzheimer's disease once it is already established but to predict with accuracy those individuals who are at risk for developing clinical symptoms. Just like in other chronic diseases, it seems clear that prevention will ultimately be the key to stopping the Alzheimer epidemic. Assuming that the most effective therapeutics will not be completely benign, it will be critical to accurately detect early changes and then be able to monitor those changes to see whether interventions have been successful. One can envision a scenario not dissimilar to the scenario that we now accept as having been so successful in tackling heart attacks and stroke: first, screening for cholesterol, blood pressure and other risk factors, followed initially by intervention that may be mild (diet, exercise) and continuing monitoring to see whether or not the risk factors have, in fact, been changed. If they haven't, medications and more aggressive strategies will be used. Ultimately, combinations of therapies will be brought to bear. All of this depends upon having excellent, presymptomatic quantitative screens for the presence of pathological changes and the ability to monitor these over time. This is the promise of identifying Alzheimer lesions in the living brain.

As potential anti-amyloid therapies are developed in a variety of venues, we will need ways of rapidly determining whether or not, and under which circumstances, these work best. Direct imaging of amyloid seems clearly the most straightforward way to do this, although other approaches are also extremely promising and may well contribute. Finally, definitive and early diagnosis important from a variety of public health and patient management issues. Even in the absence of effective therapeutics, patients and their families will benefit from a definitive and early diagnosis of risk factors.

This last point brings up one important issue. No matter how good an imaging test is, the neuroradiologist will be in no better position than the neuropathologist in determining whether or not the changes or lesions observed have resulted in cognitive impairment. Imaging of the living brain may well lead to a disassociation between the diagnosis of Alzheimer changes on radiologic imaging from Alzheimer dementia. In much the same way that a cardiologist performing an angiogram cannot predict exactly the symptoms of angina that a patient might have, the neuroradiologist should not be expected to be able to determine exactly the clinical consequences of the lesions observed. Whether the presence of lesions means the presence of "disease" can be debated. Nonetheless, as better and better imaging approaches are used, we will be able to determine brain correlates of neuropsychological processes even in "preclinical" cases (Celsis et al. 1997; Cardebat et al. 1998).

Therefore, we can anticipate a medical and potentially ethical dilemma: how should we interpret "risk factors," especially those that might have an impact on an individual's cognition and decision-making abilities, in years to come? In my opinion, the critical issue will be to distinguish between the presence of risk factors that can be directly observed by imaging and actual performance in day-to-day life events. Hopefully, the emergence of anti-Alzheimer therapeutics will grow in parallel with our ability to provide early detection of risk factors. Nonetheless, as clinicians and as a society we will need to develop models for understanding brain disease that has not "yet" developed into brain illness. Thus, successful imaging of the living brain and Alzheimer's disease may bring its share of dilemmas as well as its share of hope.

Acknowledgments

Supported by NIA AG08487, the Massachusetts Alzheimer Disease Research Center, and a Pioneer award from the Alzheimer Association.

References

Alexander GE, Chen K, Pietrini P, Rapoport SI, Reiman EM (2002) Longitudinal PET evaluation of cerebral metabolic decline in dementia: a potential outcome measure in Alzheimer's disease treatment studies. Am J Psychiat 159: 738–745

Bacskai BJ, Kajdasz ST, Christie RH, Carter C, Games D, Seubert P, Schenk D, Hyman BT (2001) Imaging of amyloid-beta deposits in brains of living mice permits direct observation of clearance of plaques with immunotherapy. Nature Med 7: 369–372

Bradley KM, O'Sullivan VT, Soper ND, Nagy Z, King EM, Smith AD, Shepstone BJ (2002) Cerebral perfusion SPET correlated with Braak pathological stage in Alzheimer's disease. Brain 125: 1772–1781

Cardebat D, Demonet JF, Puel M, Agniel A, Viallard G, Celsis P (1998) Brain correlates of memory processes in patients with dementia of Alzheimer's type: a SPECT activation study. J Cereb Blood Flow Metab 18: 457–462

Celsis P, Agniel A, Cardebat D, Demonet JF, Ousset PJ, Puel M (1997) Age related cognitive decline: a clinical entity? A longitudinal study of cerebral blood flow and memory performance. J Neurol Neurosurg Psychiat 62: 601–608

Christie RH, Bacskai BJ, Zipfel WR, Williams RM, Kajdasz ST, Webb WW, Hyman BT (2001) Growth arrest of individual senile plaques in a model of Alzheimer's disease observed by in vivo multiphoton microscopy. J Neurosci 21: 858–864

Duyckaerts, Colle MA, Dessi F, Grignon Y, Piette Y, Hauw JJ (1998) The progression of the lesions in Alzheimer disease: insights from a prospective clinicopathological study. J Neural Transm Suppl 53: 119–126

Fazekas F, Alavi A, Chawluk JB, Zimmerman RA, Hackney D, Bilaniuk L, Rosen M, Alves WM, Hurtig HI, Jamieson DG, Kushner MJ, Reivich M (1989) Comparison of CT, MR, and PET in Alzheimer's dementia and normal aging. J Nucl Med 30: 1607–1615

Fox NC, Crum WR, Scahill RI, Stevens JM, Janssen JC, Rossor MN (2001) Imaging of onset and progression of Alzheimer's disease with voxel-compression mapping of serial magnetic resonance images. Lancet 358: 201–205

Gomez-Isla T, Price JL, McKeel, Jr. DW, Morris JC, Growdon JH, Hyman BT (1996) Profound loss of layer II entorhinal cortex neurons occurs in very mild Alzheimer's disease. J Neurosci 16: 4491–4500

Gomez-Isla T, Hollister R, West H, Mui S, Growdon JH,Petersen RC, Parisi JE, Hyman BT (1997) Neuronal loss correlates with but exceeds neurofibrillary tangles in Alzheimer's disease. Ann Neurol 41: 17–24

Hock C, Golombowski S, Muller-Spahn F, Naser W, Beyreuther K, Monning U, Schenk D, Vigo-Pelfrey C, Bush AM, Moir R, Tanzi RE, Growdon JH, Nitsch RM (1998) Cerebrospinal fluid levels of amyloid precursor protein and amyloid beta-peptide in Alzheimer's disease and major depression - inverse correlation with dementia severity. Eur Neurol 39: 111–118

Jack CR Jr, Petersen RC, Xu Y, O'Brien PC, Smith GE,Ivnik RJ, Tangalos EG, Kokmen E (1998) Rate of medial temporal lobe atrophy in typical aging and Alzheimer's disease. Neurology 51: 993–999

Jack C.R Jr, Slomkowski M,Gracon S, Hoover TM, Felmlee JP, Stewart K, Xu Y, Shiung M, O'Brien PC, Cha R, Knopman D, Petersen RC (2003) MRI as a biomarker of disease progression in a therapeutic trial of milameline for AD. Neurology 60: 253–260

Jagust WJ, Seab JP, Huesman RH, Valk PE, Mathis CA, Reed BR, Coxson PC, Budinger TF (1991) Diminished glucose transport in Alzheimer's disease: dynamic PET studies. J Cereb Blood Flow Metab 11: 323–330

Killiany RJ, Gomez-Isla T, Moss M, Kikinis R, Sandor T, Jolesz F, Tanzi R, Jones K, Hyman BT, Albert MS (2000) Use of structural magnetic resonance imaging to predict who will get Alzheimer's disease. Ann Neurol 47: 430–439

Klunk WE, Wang Y, Huang GF, Debnath ML, Holt DP, Mathis CA (2001) Uncharged thioflavin-T derivatives bind to amyloid-beta protein with high affinity and readily enter the brain. Life Sci 69: 1471–1484

Klunk WE, Bacskai, BJ, Mathis CA, Kajdasz ST, McLellan ME, Frosch MP, Debnath ML, Holt DP, Wang Y, Hyman BT (2002) Imaging Abeta plaques in living transgenic mice with multi-photon microscopy and methoxy-X04, a systemically administered Congo red derivative. J Neuropathol Exp Neurol 61: 797–805

Poduslo JF, Wengenack TM, Curran GL, Wisniewski T, Sigurdsson EM, Macura SI, Borowski BJ, Jack CR Jr. (2002) Molecular targeting of Alzheimer's amyloid plaques for contrast-enhanced magnetic resonance imaging. Neurobiol Dis 11: 315–329

Schott JM, Fox NC, Frost C, Scahill RI, Janssen JC, Chan D, Jenkins R, Rossor MN (2003) Assessing the onset of structural change in familial Alzheimer's disease. Ann Neurol 53: 181–188

Sihver W, Langstrom B, Nordberg A (2000) Ligands for in vivo imaging of nicotinic receptor subtypes in Alzheimer brain. Acta Neurol Scand Suppl 176: 27–33

Sperling R, Greve D, Dale A, Killiany R, Holmes J, Rosas HD, Cocchiarella A, Firth P, Rosen B, Lake S, Lange N, Routledge C, Albert M (2002) Functional MRI detection of pharmacologically induced memory impairment. Proc Natl Acad Sci USA 99: 455–460

Thompson PM, Mega MS, Woods RP, Zoumalan CI, Lindshield CJ, Blanton RE, Moussai J, Holmes CJ, CummingsJL, Toga AW (2001) Cortical change in Alzheimer's disease detected with a disease-specific population-based brain atlas. Cereb Cortex 11: 1–16

In Vivo Imaging of Alzheimer Pathology in Transgenic Mice using Multiphoton Microscopy

Brian J. Bacskai[1], William E. Klunk[2], Gregory A. Hickey[1], Jesse Skoch[1], Stephen T. Kajdasz[1], Megan E. McLellan[1], Matthew P. Frosch[1], Manik Debnath[2], Daniel Holt[2], Yanming Wang[2], Guo-feng Huang[2], Chester A. Mathis[2], and Bradley T. Hyman[1]

Abstract

Senile plaques found in Alzheimer's disease (AD) and in transgenic mouse models of AD are comprised primarily of the amyloid-β peptide. We developed an imaging technique using multiphoton microscopy to enable both detection of amyloid-β pathology in living transgenic mice and functional results of amyloid-β deposition. We used this imaging method to characterize the in vivo kinetics of a novel amyloid-binding agent (6-OH-BTA-1, or Pittsburgh compound B, "PIB") in transgenic mice. PIB is a novel, thioflavin-T analog that stains plaques, tangles and cerebrovascular amyloid in post-mortem sections of AD brain with high sensitivity and specificity that can cross the blood-brain-barrier. Individual plaques in living transgenic mice could be detected within 1 min after i.v. injection of 2-10 mg/kg PIB. Thirty min after iv injection, the fluorescence in the parenchyma was largely diminished, whereas amyloid-β deposits remained brightly labeled. These findings suggest that PIB is a viable candidate as an in vivo amyloid imaging agent that could allow both diagnostic detection of amyloid pathology and provide a biomarker to evaluate anti-amyloid drug efficacy studies in AD. We also exploited a fluorogenic probe of oxidative stress to detect free radical generation in vivo in these mouse models that is associated specifically with dense-core, but not diffuse, amyloid-β deposits. We then extended the use of multiphoton microscopy and 2',7'-dichlorodihydrofluorescein (DCF) fluorescence to screen anti-oxidants that may serve a protective role against plaque-derived oxidative stress in an ex vivo system. These results suggest that anti-oxidant therapy may play a beneficial role in the treatment of AD.

Introduction

Alzheimer's disease (AD) is the fourth leading cause of death in industrialized societies (Katzman 1993). Presently, diagnosis is based on clinical evaluation only after a patient exhibits signs of cognitive impairments, and even this diagnosis is uncertain until postmortem examination of brain tissue. Senile plaques, comprised primarily of the amyloid-β peptide (Aβ), are one of the pathological hall-

[1] Mass General Hospital, Charlestown, Massachusetts, United States;
[2] University of Pittsburgh, PA, United States

Hyman et al.
The Living Brain and Alzheimer's Disease
©Springer-Verlag Berlin Heidelberg

marks of AD. Direct imaging of amyloid-β holds the potential to be an effective tool for diagnosis and early detection of AD (Bacskai et al.,2002a). Imaging techniques such as SPECT or PET are not typically used in the diagnosis of AD due to the lack of a specific radioligand that follows the progression of the disease. MRI can detect some gross changes in anatomy, such as hippocampal atrophy or enlargement of the lateral ventricle, however, these changes typically do not occur until cognitive impairment is already evident.

While the ability to detect senile plaques in vivo has been a goal for many years, imaging of Aβ deposits has proven difficult due to the lack of suitable contrast agents. The primary difficulty has been developing an agent that would both bind to amyloid-β specifically and cross the blood-brain barrier (BBB). Only recently have compounds for in vivo imaging of Aβ been demonstrated for PET (Zhuang et al. 2001; Bacskai et al., 2002a; Klunk et al. 2002; Mathis et al. 2002; Shoghi-Jadid et al. 2002). One promising compound, 2-(4'-methylaminophenyl)-6-hydroxy-benzothiazole (commonly referred to as Pittsburgh Compound-B or simply PIB), a derivative of thioflavin T, labels plaques, neurofibrillary tangles (NFTs), and cerebral amyloid angiopathy (CAA) in tissue sections from AD patients (Klunk et al. 2001; Mathis et al. 2002). The engineered compound also crosses the BBB, allowing peripheral administration that leads to plaque targeting in the brain.

We developed an imaging technique using multiphoton microscopy that allows us to detect fluorescent signals deep within the brain of living mice, with very high resolution. The spatial resolution is several orders of magnitude higher than is currently achievable with PET, SPECT, or MRI, and allows us to examine the microscopic morphology of individual senile plaques when appropriately labeled (Bacskai et al. 2002a). Using transgenic mouse models of AD that develop Aβ deposits as they age, we were able to image individual plaques chronically for several months (Christie et al. 2001). This detection platform also allowed us to characterize the effectiveness of an anti-amyloid-β therapy and its ability to clear individually identified plaques within living mice (Bacskai et al. 2001). Multiphoton microscopy allows us to characterize, with histochemical accuracy in living transgenic mice, the specificity, distribution, and kinetics of labeling with fluorescent compounds that target Aβ deposits (Klunk et al., 2002; Mathis et al., 2002). As an important step towards imaging Aβ deposits in humans with PIB, which is fluorescent and suitable for detection with multiphoton microscopy, we characterized the kinetics of brain entry and plaque binding in vivo in several lines of transgenic mice expressing mutant human APP (Games et al., 1995; Hsiao et al. 1996). The results demonstrate that PIB is ideally suited for detecting amyloid deposits in vivo in transgenic mice, and this finding should translate directly to successful imaging in humans.

Beyond structural detection of Aβ deposits in living mice, we also used multiphoton microscopy for functional imaging of oxidative stress associated with Aβ in vivo. Using a fluorogenic reporter, 2',7'-dichlorodihydrofluorescein (DCF), we were able to image directly the generation of free radicals associated with a specific subset of Aβ deposits in different transgenic mouse models. These results demonstrate that Aβ is a source of oxidative stress in vivo, suggesting that anit-oxidant therapy to relieve that stress may be beneficial for reduction of the cellular pathology associated with plaques. Additionally, an ex vivo system was employed to rapidly screen anti-oxidants and evaluate their efficacy in reducing the oxidative stress resulting from plaques. This screen revealed that a variety of agents were able to reduce the oxidation of DCF in tissue sections, indicating a possible therapeutic role for anti-oxidants in AD.

Results

We developed an in vivo imaging technique to detect senile plaques using multi-photon microscopy. This light microscopic technique results in images with high spatial resolution, less than 1 μm, several orders of magnitude higher than other imaging techniques like PET, SPECT and MRI (Denk et al. 1990; Bacskai et al. 2002a). The technique relies on a pulsed near infrared laser (Tsunami, Spectra Physics) to excite fluorophores, but only where the photon flux is the highest, i.e., the plane of focus. This process leads to optical sectioning similar to that achieved with confocal microscopy. This principle is illustrated in Figure 1. With confocal microscopy, a laser transmits throughout the specimen, exciting fluorescent molecules within the entire cone of illumination. The out-of-focus fluorescence is rejected with the confocal aperture, leading to optical sectioning, at the expense of exciting a large volume of fluorophores (leading to accelerated photobleaching) while discarding most of the photons. Multiphoton excitation minimizes unnecessary fluorescence excitation above and below the plane of focus, due to the requirement for high photon flux. Multiphoton excitation only occurs at the plane of focus, despite the transmission of the near infrared light above and below the plane. This effect leads to optical sectioning without the need for a confocal

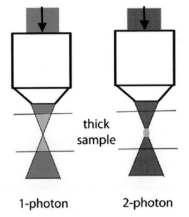

1-photon   2-photon

Fig. 1. One-photon versus two-photon excitation of fluorescence. This schematic illustrates the principle of fluorescence excitation using multiphoton microscopy. On the left is a representation of visible light excitation of a thick fluorescent sample. The sample is illuminated and excited throughout its thickness, but only the fluorescence in the plane of focus contributes to the image with confocal detection. On the right, near infrared light from a pulsed laser is used for excitation, which also illuminates the entire thickness of the sample. However, two-photon excitation occurs only at the plane of focus where the photon flux is maximal, leading to inherent optical sectioning without the need for confocal detection.

aperture. An additional advantage of multiphoton microscopy arises from this phenomen; the fluorescence emission does not have to be descanned, as is the case for confocal microscopy, but can be detected directly with optimized detectors and a shorter light path (Denk and Svoboda 1997). This process leads to greater sensitivity. Lastly, the use of near infrared light for excitation is superior to UV or visible light used in confocal microscopy because it is less harmful to living tissue, and it transmits through scattering tissue much better(Centonze and White 1998). Altogether, multiphoton microscopy is the superior choice for microscopic detection of fluorescence in thick, living tissue (Williams et al. 2001).

The principle disadvantage of multiphoton microscopy over other imaging techniques is the need to gain access to the brain in living animals. This requirement involves an invasive procedure, removing the scalp and most of the bone over the cortex. Our current surgical procedure involves removing a large circular portion of the skull and replacing it with a glass coverslip that is cemented into place (Mathis et al. 2002; Fig. 2).After this surgery, microscopy can be per-

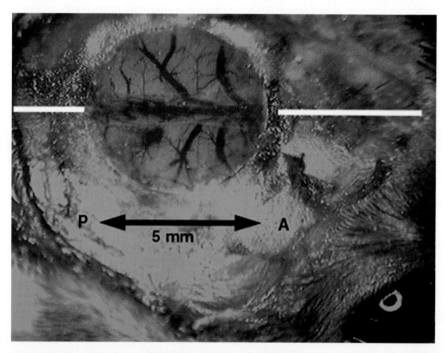

Fig. 2. Cranial window for chronic in vivo imaging. This photograph shows a freshly implanted cranial window in a living transgenic mouse. The horizontal white line marks the midline, with the anterior portion of the head to the right. A 5-mm craniotomy was made, spanning the midline. In this case, the dura was carefully reflected from each side, excluding the region directly above the sagittal sinus. Sterile PBS was applied to the surface of the brain, and a 5-mm glass coverslip was floated on top. A mixture of cyanoacrylate adhesive and dental cement was used to adhere the coverslip to the adjacent surface of the skull. After cementing the coverslip, the animal was allowed to recover, without suturing the scalp back in place, and survived without any apparent discomfort.

formed through the cranial window in the live mouse. After imaging, the mouse can recover and live comfortably with the coverslip in place for months, allowing chronic imaging of the brain within single animals.

With the imaging techniques in place, we are able to detect senile plaques within the brains of transgenic mouse models that overexpress various mutant forms of human APP. These animals develop senile plaques and cerebreovascular amyloid angiopathy (CAA) as they age (Games et al. 1995; Hsiao et al. 1996). We used these animals to characterize the kinetics of brain entry of a systemically administered compound that would be a good candidate for PET imaging in humans, Pittsburgh compound B, or "PIB." PET imaging requires radiolabeling of the tracer compound, limiting the time window for use due to the short half-life of the radioactive molecule. Therefore, an optimal time for imaging after systemic administration needs to be determined, bracketed by large quantities of unbound tracer soon after injection, and loss of signal late after injection. The kinetics of specific labeling and non-specific clearance must therefore be characterized and optimized for each radiolabeled probe. Using multiphoton microscopy, we capitalized on the intrinsic fluorescence of PIB and characterized the kinetics of brain entry and clearance in transgenic mouse models of AD. The specific binding of PIB to Aβ deposits could be determined with very high spatial resolution, and confirmed with histochemistry. Figure 3 shows PIB labeling of CAA and parenchymal plaques within an imaging volume of a living transgenic mouse, 60 min after iv injection of 2 mg/kg of the compound. The Aβ deposits were detected with sub-micron resolution and show high contrast labeling with little non-specific binding to other structures.

For real-time kinetic determinations, an intravenous line was implanted into a tail vein of an anesthetized mouse. Multiphoton microscopy was used to image a volume of the cortex over time, resulting in four-dimensional data collection. Before injection, little autofluorescence was detectable within the brain. At time zero, a bolus of 2-10 mg/kg PIB was injected and was detectable within the cerebral vasculature within seconds. Within one minute, the fluorescent compound was observed to cross the blood-brain-barrier (BBB) and enter the parenchyma. Large vessels with CAA were labeled almost immediately with the compound. Parenchymal Aβ deposits took slightly longer to become labeled and 10-20 min to become labeled completely. In the meantime, intravascular and unbound parenchymal fluorescence was markedly reduced from its peak on a time scale of minutes. Figure 4 illustrates the temporal dynamics of brain entry, labeling and brain exit. Each trace represents the mean fluorescence intensity over time from blood vessels with and without CAA, and parenchymal volumes with and without senile plaques. Note that the Aβ deposits were labeled quickly and remained labeled, whereas non-specific fluorescence decreased rapidly in areas devoid of amyloid. These results demonstrate, in real time, that systemically injected PIB crosses the BBB and labels amyloid-β deposits. The unbound dye clears rapidly from the vasculature and parenchyma. Altogether, the kinetics and specificity of PIB in the transgenic mouse models suggest that this compound should be an excellent candidate for imaging Aβ deposits in humans.

While these results strengthen and confirm the utility of PIB for Aβ detection in vivo, multiphoton microscopy was also used for functional imaging in the

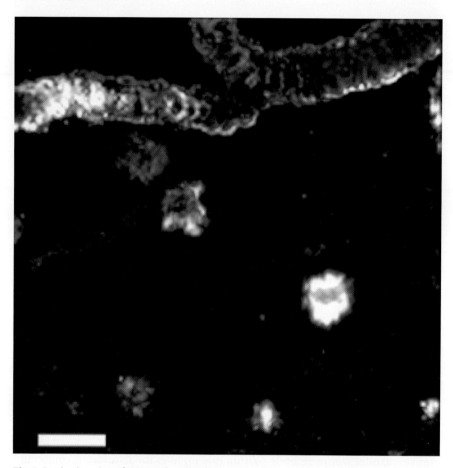

Fig. 3. In vivo imaging of CAA and senile plaques after intravenous administration of PIB. This is a maximum intensity projection of a volume of the brain of a living Tg2576 mouse (20-month-old) 60 min after iv injection of 2 mg/kg PIB. The imaging volume was acquired with multiphoton excitation at 750 nm, and fluorescence emission centered at 440 nm. Along the top of the image is a blood vessel containing cerebral amyloid angiopathy. Numerous parenchymal Aβ deposits can be seen as well. Scale bar = 50μm.

transgenic mice. We took advantage of the availability of a fluorogenic probe for oxidative stress to determine, for the first time, whether oxidative stress occurs in models of AD in vivo (McLellan et al. 2003). The role of oxidative stress in AD has been hotly debated for years, with some investigators suggesting it is a cause of the disease (Yan et al. 1995; Nunomura et al. 2000; Pratico et al. 2001), whereas others argue that it is the result of plaque deposition, further exacerbating the disease (Good et al. 1996; Smith et al. 1996; Wong et al. 2001). The data concerning the relevance of oxidative stress in AD result from in vitro studies describing the contributions from synthetic peptides (Hensley et al. 1994; Mattson and Goodman 1995; Keller et al. 1997) or from immunohistochemical determinations of

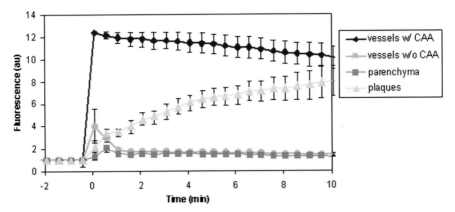

Fig. 4. Time-course of brain entry, clearance, and amyloid labeling with PIB. A 20-month-old Tg2576 mouse was imaged using multiphoton microscopy. At t=0, a bolus i.V. injection of 2 mg/kg PIB was administered and detected within the cerebral vasculature. CAA was labeled rapidly whereas parenchymal plaques required several minutes to be labeled completely. Most of the unbound fluorescence from the vasculature and parenchyma was quickly cleared. Each point is the average of at least three regions of interest from within the imaging volume. These results demonstrate that PIB crosses the blood-brain barrier quickly, enters the parenchyma and labels amyloid deposits specifically.

proteins or lipids downstream of oxidative damage in tissue sections from AD cases (Montine et al. 1997; Sayre et al. 1997; Leutner et al. 2000). Using transgenic mouse models of AD and multiphoton microscopy, we imaged a fluorescent reporter of oxidative stress, 2',7'-dichlorodihydrofluorescein (DCF), in vivo (LeBel et al. 1992). This reporter is non-fluorescent in its reduced form, but upon oxidation it becomes brightly fluorescent. Topical application of this probe to the surface of the cortex in a living transgenic mouse led to a specific localization of fluorescence within the brain. Figure 5 demonstrates that DCF led to high-contrast fluorescent images of dense-core senile plaques in the brain. CAA was also detectable by DCF fluorescence. No other fluorescence was observed in the brain, despite the availability of reactive dye throughout the imaging volume. After imaging, thioflavine S was topically applied, and the same brain volume was imaged. In this case, thioflavine S labeled Aβ deposits that were previously identified with DCF fluorescence (Fig. 5B). Post-mortem immunohistochemistry was used to determine that diffuse Aβ deposits were also present within the imaging volume but did not lead to oxidation of DCF. Therefore, only a subset of senile plaques in the mouse model leads to the generation of free radicals. The thioflavine S-positive, dense-core plaques are also the same subset of plaques associated with dystrophic neurites (Masliah et al. 1990; Knowles et al. 1998, 1999) and neuronal loss (Urbanc et al. 2002), so it is intriguing to speculate about a correlation between these two events.

To determine if live cells associated with dense-core plaques or the plaques themselves were responsible for oxidation of DCF, we performed a similar analysis of oxidative stress in an ex vivo preparation, using tissue sections. The 40-μm

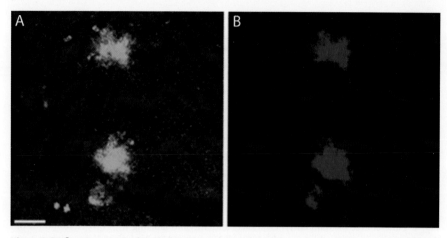

Fig. 5. DCF fluorescence is observed on dense-core plaques in vivo. The fluorescent reporter of oxidative stress, DCF, was topically applied to the cortex of a living 18-month-old Tg2576 mouse for 30 min and then washed with PBS. Multiphoton microscopy was used to detect fluorescence within the first 300 μm of the cortex under the cranial window. Fluorescence was observed from structures that appeared to be senile plaques (A) and CAA (not shown). After imaging, the coverslip was removed, and 0.005% thioflavin S was topically applied to the brain for 20 min. The same volumes of the brain were imaged, revealing that the DCF-labeled structures were dense-core plaques, as defined by thioflavin S staining (B). Scale bar = 20μm.

thick, fixed sections from transgenic mouse brain have no live cells, but abundant Aβ deposits. Incubation of the tissue with non-fluorescent DCF led to the appearance of fluorescence that was specifically localized to dense-core plaques, detectable with multiphoton microscopy, identical to the observations in vivo. This result demonstrates that the Aβ deposits themselves are responsible for the oxidation of DCF and not the surrounding microglia, neurons, or astrocytes. This approach also allows rapid determinations of DCF fluorescence and screening of anti-oxidants capable of reducing the oxidative stress that is associated with dense-core plaques. Identification of effective anti-oxidants could lead to therapies useful for preventing or treating AD in human patients. Therefore, we evaluated the ability of two known anti-oxidants, *N-tert*-butyl-α-phenylnitrone (PBN; Behl et al. 1994; Socci et al.,1995) and Ginkgo biloba extract EGb761 (Luo 2001; Bastianetto and Quirion 2002; Doraiswamy 2002; Grundman and Delaney 2002; Zimmermann et al. 2002) on their ability to prevent or reduce the plaque-specific oxidation of DCF. Figure 6 indicates that both of these compounds are capable of reducing the generation of fluorescent DCF elicited by dense-core plaques in the tissue sections. For PBN, at 100 μM, fluorescence was reduced by 65% (McLellan et al. 2003); for Ginkgo biloba extract EGb761 at 0.5 mg/ml, fluorescence was reduced by 58%. In each of these determinations, six tissue sections from at least three mice were used. These results suggest that each of these anti-oxidants is suitable for testing for its ability to prevent or halt the deleterious effects of dense-core senile plaques in animal models and may lead to an optimized anti-oxidant therapy suitable for use in humans.

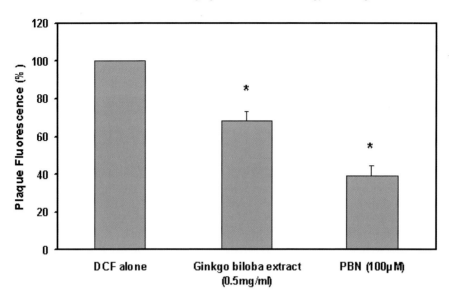

Fig. 6. An **ex vivo** assay for oxidative stress in AD tissue reveals effective anti-oxidant treatments. These data represent quantitative determinations of DCF fluorescence in fixed sections of tissue from Tg2576 mouse brain. Tissue sections were pre-treated with the anti-oxidants PBN (100 μM) and Ginkgo biloba extract EGb761 (0.5 mg/ml) for 1 hr in PBS. DCF (200 μM) was added in the continued presence of the anti-oxidants for an additional 60 min. After washing with PBS, the sections were mounted in aqueous media and imaged using multiphoton microscopy. The fluorescence of DCF from individual dense-core plaques was measured using Scion Image software (Scioncorp). After imaging, the coverslips were removed, and 0.005% thioflavin S was added to the tissue sections for 20 min. The sections were coverslipped again and re-imaged using multiphoton microscopy. A background corrected ratio of the fluorescence of DCF from each plaque to the fluorescence from thioflavin S for that plaque was calculated and compared to the fluorescence ratio of DCF-treated slides that did not receive anti-oxidant treatment. Each bar in the graph represents the mean ± standard. error of at least 50 plaques from n=3 mice. The ratios were normalized to a value of 100% for DCF alone-treated tissue. These results demonstrate that the oxidation of DCF can be partially prevented by both PBN and Ginkgo biloba extract, suggesting that each anti-oxidant may be suitable for anti-oxidant therapy in AD.

Discussion

In this report, we present results using multiphoton microscopy for anatomical and functional imaging of senile plaques in living transgenic mouse models of AD. Multiphoton microscopy is a light microscopic imaging technique that produces high resolution images through thick, intact biological samples (Denk et al. 1990; Williams et al. 2001). It is superior to confocal imaging, using visible light excitation in intact brain, and has a spatial resolution several orders of magnitude higher than conventional imaging techniques like PET, SPECT, or MRI (Bacskai et al. 2002a). The major drawbacks of multiphoton microscopy for brain imaging are the reduced volume of brain that can be imaged (albeit at very high resolution) and the need for an invasive procedure to gain access to the brain. We have shown previously that this technique is capable of detecting individual plaques chronically in living mice (Christie et al., 2001) and that anti- Aβ therapies can lead to clearance of existing plaques with single treatments (Bacskai et al. 2001). We have also explored the mechanism of action of immunotherapy, as a step towards optimizing this approach for successful use in human patients (Bacskai et al. 2002b).

Using animal models of plaque development, we have characterized several novel contrast reagents, accelerating their development and application as tools for use in diagnostic imaging with PET in humans(Klunk et al. 2002; Mathis et al. 2002). The current work utilizes the high temporal resolution afforded by multiphoton microscopy to measure the kinetics of a promising PET probe, PIB. We have shown that PIB enters the cerebral circulation rapidly after iv injection, crosses the BBB quickly, and labels CAA within seconds. After entering the parenchyma, plaques are labeled within minutes. Unbound dye is rapidly cleared from the circulation and the parenchyma, within 20 minutes. PIB that is bound to Aβ deposits remains bound for long times; it is detectable for up to three days in our hands. Altogether, these kinetics describe desirable characteristics for a PET probe that targets Aβ in vivo, demonstrating that PIB is a great candidate for diagnostic imaging of Aβ in humans.

We have also shown that multiphoton microscopy is ideally suited for functional imaging in brains of living transgenic mice. Using the fluorogenic reporter DCF, we localized the source of oxidative stress from parenchymal deposits to a subset of senile plaques (McLellan et al. 2003). Dense-core plaques (histochemically defined by thioflavine S staining) but not diffuse plaques were sources of oxidative activity in the brains of transgenic mice. This subset of Aβ deposits is associated with dystrophic neuronal processes and neuronal death in the mouse models, suggesting a possible correlation between the excess oxidative capacity of these Aβ deposits and neuronal impairment. CAA also led to an increase in fluorescence from DCF, demonstrating that it, too, is a source of free radicals. Using an ex vivo assay, we evaluated the ability of the anti-oxidants PBN and Ginkgo biloba extract EGb761 to inhibit the oxidation of DCF by dense-core Aβ deposits and found that both compounds were effective. Therefore, this assay should be well-suited to quickly screen anti-oxidants that may translate to effective therapies to prevent or reduce the oxidative damage resulting from senile plaques in AD.

Acknowledgements

This work supported by NIH: AG08487 (BTH), AG18402 (CM), AG01039 (WEK), AG20226 (WEK), AG15453 (BTH), EB00768 (BJB), AG020570 (BJB), the Alzheimer Association: Pioneer Award (BTH), IIRG-95-076 (WEK), TLL-01-3381 (WEK) and NIRG-00-2355 (YW), and ISOA/AFAR: 210304 (YW). We thank Drs. D. Games and D. Schenk, Elan Pharmaceuticals, for access to PDAPP mice.

References

Bacskai BJ, Kajdasz ST, Christie RH, Carter C, Games D, Seubert P, Schenk D, Hyman BT (2001) Imaging of amyloid-beta deposits in brains of living mice permits direct observation of clearance of plaques with immunotherapy. Nature Med 7:369-372

Bacskai BJ, Klunk WE, Mathis CA, Hyman BT (2002a) Imaging amyloid-beta deposits in vivo. J Cereb Blood Flow Metab 22:1035-1041

Bacskai BJ, Kajdasz ST, McLellan ME, Games D, Seubert P, Schenk D, Hyman BT (2002b) Non-Fc-mediated mechanisms are involved in clearance of amyloid-beta in vivo by immunotherapy. J Neurosci 22:7873-7878

Bastianetto S, Quirion R (2002) EGb 761 is a neuroprotective agent against beta-amyloid toxicity. Cell Mol Biol (Noisy-le-grand) 48:693-697

Behl C, Davis JB, Lesley R, Schubert D (1994) Hydrogen peroxide mediates amyloid beta protein toxicity. Cell 77:817-827

Centonze VE, White JG (1998) Multiphoton excitation provides optical sections from deeper within scattering specimens than confocal imaging. Biophys J 75:2015-2024

Christie RH, Bacskai BJ, Zipfel WR, Williams RM, Kajdasz ST, Webb WW, Hyman BT (2001) Growth arrest of individual senile plaques in a model of Alzheimer's disease observed by in vivo multiphoton microscopy. J Neurosci 21:858-864

Denk W, Svoboda K (1997) Photon upmanship: why multiphoton imaging is more than a gimmick. Neuron 18:351-357

Denk W, Strickler JH, Webb WW (1990) Two-photon laser scanning fluorescence microscopy. Science 248:73-76

Doraiswamy PM (2002) Non-cholinergic strategies for treating and preventing Alzheimer's disease. CNS Drugs 16:811-824

Games D, Adams D, Alessandrini R, Barbour R, Berthelette P, Blackwell C, Carr T, Clemens J, Donaldson T, Gillespie F, Guido T, Hagoplan S, Johnson-Wood K, Kahn K, Lee M, Leibowitz P, Lieberburg I, Little S, Masliah E, McConlogue L, Montoya-Zavala M, Mucke L, Paganini L, Penniman E, Power M, Schenk D, Seubert P, Snyder B, Soriano F, Tan H, Vitale J, Wadsworth S, Wolozin B, Zhao J (1995) Alzheimer-type neuropathology in transgenic mice overexpressing V717F beta-amyloid precursor protein. Nature 373:523-527

Good PF, Werner P, Hsu A, Olanow CW, Perl DP (1996) Evidence of neuronal oxidative damage in Alzheimer's disease. Am J Pathol 149:21-28

Grundman M, Delaney P (2002) Antioxidant strategies for Alzheimer's disease. Proc Nutr Soc 61:191-202

Hensley K, Carney JM, Mattson MP, Aksenova M, Harris M, Wu JF, Floyd RA, Butterfield DA (1994) A model for beta-amyloid aggregation and neurotoxicity based on free radical generation by the peptide: relevance to Alzheimer disease. Proc Natl Acad Sci USA 91:3270-3274

Hsiao K, Chapman P, Nilsen S, Eckman C, Harigaya Y, Younkin S, Yang F, Cole G (1996) Correlative memory deficits, Abeta elevation, and amyloid plaques in transgenic mice. Science 274:99-102

Katzman R (1993) Education and the prevalence of dementia and Alzheimer's disease. . Neurology 43:13-20

Keller JN, Pang Z, Geddes JW, Begley JG, Germeyer A, Waeg G, Mattson MP (1997) Impairment of glucose and glutamate transport and induction of mitochondrial oxidative stress and dysfunction in synaptosomes by amyloid beta-peptide: role of the lipid peroxidation product 4- hydroxynonenal. J Neurochem 69:273-284

Klunk WE, Wang Y, Huang GF, Debnath ML, Holt DP, Mathis CA (2001) Uncharged thioflavin-T derivatives bind to amyloid-beta protein with high affinity and readily enter the brain. Life Sci 69:1471-1484

Klunk WE, Bacskai BJ, Mathis CA, Kajdasz ST, McLellan ME, Frosch MP, Debnath ML, Holt DP, Wang Y, Hyman BT (2002) Imaging Abeta plaques in living transgenic mice with multiphoton microscopy and methoxy-X04, a systemically administered Congo red derivative. J Neuropathol Exp Neurol 61:797-805

Knowles RB, Gomez-Isla T, Hyman BT (1998) Abeta associated neuropil changes: correlation with neuronal loss and dementia. J Neuropathol Exp Neurol 57:1122-1130

Knowles RB, Wyart C, Buldyrev SV, Cruz L, Urbanc B, Hasselmo ME, Stanley HE, Hyman BT (1999) Plaque-induced neurite abnormalities: implications for disruption of neural networks in Alzheimer's disease. Proc Natl Acad Sci USA 96:5274-5279

LeBel CP, Ischiropoulos H, Bondy SC (1992) Evaluation of the probe 2',7'-dichlorofluorescin as an indicator of reactive oxygen species formation and oxidative stress. Chem Res Toxicol 5:227-231

Leutner S, Czech C, Schindowski K, Touchet N, Eckert A, Muller WE (2000) Reduced antioxidant enzyme activity in brains of mice transgenic for human presenilin-1 with single or multiple mutations. Neurosci Lett 292:87-90

Luo Y (2001) Ginkgo biloba neuroprotection: Therapeutic implications in Alzheimer's disease. J Alzheimers Dis 3:401-407

Masliah E, Terry RD, Mallory M, Alford M, Hansen LA (1990) Diffuse plaques do not accentuate synapse loss in Alzheimer's disease. Am J Pathol 137:1293-1297

Mathis CA, Bacskai BJ, Kajdasz ST, McLellan ME, Frosch MP, Hyman BT, Holt DP, Wang Y, Huang GF, Debnath ML, Klunk WE (2002) A lipophilic thioflavin-T derivative for positron emission tomography (PET) imaging of amyloid in brain. Bioorg Med Chem Lett 12:295-298

Mattson MP, Goodman Y (1995) Different amyloidogenic peptides share a similar mechanism of neurotoxicity involving reactive oxygen species and calcium. Brain Res 676:219-224

McLellan ME, Kajdasz ST, Hyman BT, Bacskai BJ (2003) In vivo imaging of reactive oxygen species specifically associated with thioflavine S-positive amyloid plaques by multiphoton microscopy. Journal of Neuroscience In Press.

Montine KS, Olson SJ, Amarnath V, Whetsell WO, Jr., Graham DG, Montine TJ (1997) Immunohistochemical detection of 4-hydroxy-2-nonenal adducts in Alzheimer's disease is associated with inheritance of APOE4. Am J Pathol 150:437-443

Nunomura A, Perry G, Pappolla MA, Friedland RP, Hirai K, Chiba S, Smith MA (2000) Neuronal oxidative stress precedes amyloid-beta deposition in Down syndrome. J Neuropathol Exp Neurol 59:1011-1017

Pratico D, Uryu K, Leight S, Trojanoswki JQ, Lee VM (2001) Increased lipid peroxidation precedes amyloid plaque formation in an animal model of Alzheimer amyloidosis. J Neurosci 21:4183-4187

Sayre LM, Zelasko DA, Harris PL, Perry G, Salomon RG, Smith MA (1997) 4-Hydroxynonenal-derived advanced lipid peroxidation end products are increased in Alzheimer's disease. J Neurochem 68:2092-2097

Shoghi-Jadid K, Small GW, Agdeppa ED, Kepe V, Ercoli LM, Siddarth P, Read S, Satyamurthy N, Petric A, Huang SC, Barrio JR (2002) Localization of neurofibrillary tangles and beta-amyloid plaques in the brains of living patients with Alzheimer disease. Am J Geriatr Psychiatry 10:24-35

Smith MA, Perry G, Richey PL, Sayre LM, Anderson VE, Beal MF, Kowall N (1996) Oxidative damage in Alzheimer's. Nature 382:120-121

Socci DJ, Crandall BM, Arendash GW (1995) Chronic antioxidant treatment improves the cognitive performance of aged rats. Brain Res 693:88-94

Urbanc B, Cruz L, Le R, Sanders J, Ashe KH, Duff K, Stanley HE, Irizarry MC, Hyman BT (2002) Neurotoxic effects of thioflavin S-positive amyloid deposits in transgenic mice and Alzheimer's disease. Proc Natl Acad Sci USA 99:13990-13995

Williams RM, Zipfel WR, Webb WW (2001) Multiphoton microscopy in biological research. Curr Opin Chem Biol 5:603-608

Wong A, Luth HJ, Deuther-Conrad W, Dukic-Stefanovic S, Gasic-Milenkovic J, Arendt T, Munch G (2001) Advanced glycation endproducts co-localize with inducible nitric oxide synthase in Alzheimer's disease. Brain Res 920:32-40

Yan SD, Yan SF, Chen X, Fu J, Chen M, Kuppusamy P, Smith MA, Perry G, Godman GC, Nawroth P, Zweier JL, Stern D (1995) Non-enzymatically glycated tau in Alzheimer's disease induces neuronal oxidant stress resulting in cytokine gene expression and release of amyloid beta-peptide. Nature Med 1:693-699

Zhuang ZP, Kung MP, Hou C, Plossl K, Skovronsky D, Gur TL, Trojanowski JQ, Lee VM, Kung HF (2001) IBOX(2-(4'-dimethylaminophenyl)-6-iodobenzoxazole): a ligand for imaging amyloid plaques in the brain. Nucl Med Biol 28:887-894

Zimmermann M, Colciaghi F, Cattabeni F, Di Luca M (2002) Ginkgo biloba extract: from molecular mechanisms to the treatment of Alzhelmer's disease. Cell Mol Biol (Noisy-le-grand) 48:613-623

In Vivo Magnetic Resonance of Amyloid Plaques in Alzheimer's Disease Model Mice

Einar M. Sigurdsson[1,3], *Youssef Zaim Wadghiri*[4,5], *Marcin Sadowski*[2],
James I. Elliott[6], *Yongsheng Li*[2], *Henrieta Scholtzova*[2], *Cheuk Ying Tang*[7],
Gilbert Aguinaldo[7], *Karen Duff*[8], *Daniel H. Turnbull*[3,4,5],
Thomas Wisniewski[1,2,3]*

Summary

A key feature of Alzheimer's disease (AD) is the deposition of the amyloid β (Aβ) as neuritic plaques in the brain. Transgenic mice overexpressing mutant amyloid precursor protein (APP), or both mutant APP and presenilin-1 (APP-PS1), develop Aβ plaques similar to AD patients and are currently the most widely used models of AD. The definitive diagnosis of AD still requires post-mortem examination. We have developed a novel method for the detection of Aβ plaques in the brains of AD model transgenic mice using magnetic resonance micro-imaging (μMRI). Our method is dependent on ligands that bind to AD amyloid lesions, allowing their detection by μMRI. These ligands are Aβ1-40 peptides, magnetically labeled with either gadolinium (Gd) or monocrystalline iron oxide nanoparticles (MION). When these are systemically injected with mannitol to transiently open the blood-brain barrier, we are able to detect the majority of amyloid lesions. The number of lesions detected by μMRI showed a statistically significant correlation with the Aβ burden determined by histology. This approach, with additional development, may be used to detect amyloid lesions in humans. Similar methods may also be used to image other conformational neurodegenerative disorders.

Introduction

Currently, the definitive diagnosis of AD requires post-mortem examination. The presence of amyloid-β (Aβ) plaques, neurofibrillary tangles and cell loss in various brain regions, in conjunction with dementia, are the hallmarks of AD. It is commonly thought that the disease progresses for years or even decades before clinical symptoms become evident (Morris 1999; Price and Morris 1999). An early diagnosis of AD would be very useful, especially when effective treatments are available to slow its progression. Studies of biological markers for AD in body fluids have been disappointing, but the use of novel, in vivo imaging techniques

Department of Psychiatry[1], Neurology[2], Pathology[3], and Radiology[4], and Skirball Institute of Biommolecular Medicine[5], 550 First Avenue, New York NY 10016, and Department of Molecular Biophysics and Biochemistry[6], Yale University, New Haven CT and Departments of Radiology and Psychiatry[7], Mount Sinai School of Medicine, New York NY and Nathan Kline Institute[8], New York University, Orangeburg, NY may provide a sensitive method for diagnosing AD in its early stages. Amyloid plaques are found extracellularly and are much larger than the mostly intracellular neurofibrillary tangles and may therefore provide the most accessible target for imaging.

A number of different transgenic mouse lines have been developed to model Alzheimer's disease (AD). Mice overexpressing either mutant amyloid precursor protein (APP), or both mutant APP and presenilin-1 (APP/PS1), develop extensive Aβ plaques, one of the key features of AD (Holcomb et al. 1998; Hsiao et al. 1996).

These mice are being widely used to test therapies of AD that clear amyloid (Janus et al. 2000; Morgan et al. 2001; Schenk et al. 1999); hence, we chose these mouse models for our imaging studies. Prior in vitro studies have shown that radiolabeled Aβ binds to Aβ plaques (Maggio et al. 1992). More recent studies have shown that radiolabeled Aβ derivatives (Lee et al. 2002; Mackic et al. 2002; Wengenack et al. 2000a) or other radioactive probes that bind to β (Marshall et al. 2002; Skovronsky et al. 2000) allow the visualization of Aβ plaques following autoradiography of tissue sections. The development of a contrast agent that selectively binds to β might enable plaque detection with sufficient temporal, spatial and contrast resolution using in vivo μMRI in AD transgenic mice. We have tagged Aβ1-40, an Aβ peptide with high binding affinity for itself and other Aβ peptides found in AD plaques (Jarrett and Lansbury Jr. 1993), with two paramagnetic MRI contrast agents: gadolinium-diethylenetriaminepentaacetic acid (Gd-DTPA), and monocrystalline iron oxide nanoparticles (MION). Our results show that these two magnetically labeled ligands, Gd-DTPA-Aβ1-40 and Aβ1-40-coated MION particles, can be used to detect Aβ plaques in the brains of both APP and APP/PS1 transgenic mice after intravascular co-injection with mannitol to transiently open the blood-brain barrier (BBB).

Methods

Magnetically Labeled Peptides

Aβ1-40 with and without a metal chelating arm were synthesized on a ABI 430A peptide synthesizer using standard protocols for tBOC (tert-butyloxycarbonyl) chemistry. The chelating arm, DTPA, was attached to the amino terminus of the peptide as the final step of synthesis. The peptides were cleaved from the resins using hydrofluoric acid, and purification was performed by high pressure liquid chromatography (HPLC) on a Vydac C18 preparative column, 2.5 x 30 cm (Vydac Separations, Hesperia, CA), using linear gradients from 0-70% of acetonitrile in 0.1% trifluoroacetic acid. Gadolinium (Gd) was chelated to the DTPA-Aβ peptide using Gd (III) chloride hexahydrate (Aldrich, Milwaukee WI, 27,852-1) with a 24-hour incubation in water at pH 7.0. Mass spectroscopy of HPLC purified Gd-DTPA-Aβ1-40 gave a mass of 4975.76, in agreement with the expected mass of 4976.6. MIONs were obtained from the Center for Molecular Imaging Research (Massachusetts General Hospital, Boston, MA) as a brownish, stock solution containing 12.05 mg Fe/ml. Each MION particle contains an average of 2,064 Fe molecules (Weissleder et al. 2000). For injection into each mouse, 300 µg of dex-tran-coated MION particles (15.8 µl of stock solution) was adsorbed with 120 µg of Aβ1-40 in a volume of 120 µl of H2O by overnight mixing at 4°C (Moore et al. 1997; Shen et al. 1993; Xu et al. 1998).

Magnetic Resonance Micro-imaging (µMRI)

µMRI experiments were performed on either a SMIS console interfaced to a 7 Tesla (T) horizontal bore magnet equipped with 250 mT/m actively shielded gradients (Magnex Scientific, Abingdon UK) or a 9.4T, 89-mm vertical bore system operating at a proton frequency of 400 MHz (Bruker Instruments) with a gradient insert having an internal diameter (ID) of 75 mm, capable of generating a maximum of 100 mT/m. Preliminary imaging experiments were performed to assess the relaxivity effects of unlabeled, Gd-labeled and MION-labeled peptides in a water solution (Fig. 1).

For in vivo µMRI the mice were initially anesthetized with isoflurane (5%) in air, and anesthesia was maintained with 1.5% isoflurane in air (2 l/min flow rate). The rectal temperature and respiratory rate of each mouse were monitored throughout the scan. A custom saddle coil (ID = 22 mm) was incorporated into the holding device, and a tooth bar was used to fix the head in a reproducible and stationary position during data acquisition. As in the ex vivo imaging protocol, coronal brain image slices were acquired for each mouse using a T2-weighted spin echo sequence (TE = 30 ms; TR = 2 s; 78 µm x 78 µm in-plane resolution; 500 µm slice thickness; total imaging time = 120min) or a T2*- weighted gradient echo sequence (TE = 15 ms; TR = 1.5 s; 78 µm x 78 µm in-plane resolution; 250 µm slice thickness; total imaging time = 59 minutes) was used to increase the susceptibility contrast of the magnetically labelled Aβ. After euthanasia brains of in vivo-imaged mice were reimaged using the ex vivo protocol.

Mice and Contrast Agent Injection

Gd-DTPA-Aβ1-40 was prepared before each administration by suspending 400 µg in 100 µl water and dissolving immediately before infusion with a solution of 15% mannitol in PBS (600 µl), in order to temporarily open the BBB (Chi et al. 1997; Siegal et al. 2000). This preparation was injected directly into the common carotid artery at a rate of 0.25ml/kg/sec. This rate is below that which causes hypertensive opening of the BBB, but gives optimal BBB disruption without neurotoxicity (Chi et al. 1997; Cosolo et al. 1989). This dosage of Gd-DTPA-Aβ1-40 represents a much smaller dose of Gd- DTPA per body weight than is used in a typical human clinical study (0.2 ml/kg). This human dose, scaled to the mouse's body weight, corresponds to 472 µg of Gd, whereas we used 12.6 µg of Gd per mouse (400 µg x 157.25/4976), or approximately 3% of the human dose.

In other experiments, MION-Aβ1-40 was used as the contrast agent. In this case each mouse received 300 µg of MION particles, on to which 120 µg of Aβ1-40 was absorbed. The dosage of MION reported in human studies has ranged bet-

1. Synthesis and characterization of Aβ-specific ligands for μMRI:

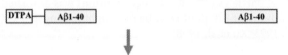

2. MR contrast Agent Tagging:

Chelation: **Absorption:**

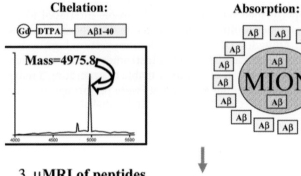

3. μMRI of peptides

Gd-DTPA-Aβ1-40   Aβ1-40   MION-Aβ1-40

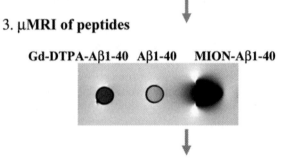

4. *In vivo* intra-carotid injection, of peptides with mannitol

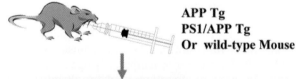

APP Tg
PS1/APP Tg
Or wild-type Mouse

5. In vivo μMRI or μMRI of extracted, whole brains

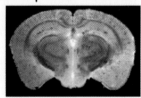

Fig. 1. Schematic representation of the synthesis and characterization of the two Aβ-specific-binding ligands for μMRI. Aβ1-40 was first synthesized with and without the chelating group, DPTA, on its amino terminus, followed by HPLC purification. The DPTA-Aβ1-40 was then used to chelate Gd, the Gd-DPTA-Aβ1-40 was repurified by HPLC and the expected mass was verified by mass spectroscopy. Each DPTA-Aβ1-40 chelates a single Gd ion. Mass spectroscopy of the HPLC-purified Gd-DTPA-Aβ1-40 gave a mass of 4975.76, in good agreement with expected mass of 4976.6. Alternatively, the Aβ1- 40 was absorbed onto MION. μMRI of the Gd-DTPA-Aβ1-40 and MION-Aβ1-40 at the same concentrations used for injection showed the expected T2-weighted signal loss and susceptibility effects of Gd-DTPA and MION, whereas unlabeled Aβ1-40 showed no T2-weighted signal effect. The Aβ1-40 alone, Gd-DPTA- Aβ1-40 or MION-Aβ1-40 were then injected with or without 15% mannitol in vivo into the carotid artery of wild-type, APP or APP/PS1 transgenic mice. Six hours after injection the mouse brains were imaged in vivo or ex vivo with μMRI.

---

ween 1.1 and 2.6 mgFe/kg (Bellin et al. 2000; Enochs et al. 1999; Harisinghani et al. 1997, 1999, 2001; Nguyen et al. 1999); hence, the mice received a substantially higher dose. Immediately before injection into the common carotid artery, MION-Aβ1-40 was mixed with 600 μl of 15% mannitol in PBS. Both Gd-DTPA-Aβ1-40 and MION-Aβ1-40 were co-injected with mannitol into six-month-old APP/PS1 transgenic mice, 15- to 16-month-old APP transgenic mice, as well as age-matched, non-transgenic controls. A number of additional control experiments were performed, injecting Gd-DTPA-Aβ1-40 without mannitol, Gd-DTPA with mannitol but without Aβ1-40, or no injection. Six hours after intra-carotid injection, the mice were imaged in vivo. Six hours was chosen as a time point since our own and other studies using 125I-Aβ1-40 have shown that the time of maximum AD plaque labeling following systemic injections, with minimal non-specific labeling of blood vessels, is between four and six hours (Mackic et al. 2002; Wengenack et al. 2000a).

Histology

Following imaging, the brains were placed in 2% DMSO/20% glycerol in 0.1 M phosphate buffer, pH 7.4, overnight. Subsequently, coronal sections (40 μm) were cut and serial sections at 0.2 mm intervals were saved for histological analysis of 1) 6E10, 2) Congo red or 3) Mallory stained sections. 6E10 (Kim et al. 1990) recognizes Ab. Congo red staining was performed to distinguish amyloid from preamyloid Ab immunoreactive deposits. The Mallory iron-staining method enabled us to detect MION particles associated with the Aβ plaques. The series were placed in ethylene glycol cryoprotectant and stored at -20°C until used.

Amyloid Burden Quantitation

Immunohistochemistry of tissue sections was quantified with a Bioquant stereology image analysis system (R&M Biometrics Inc., Nashville, TN) using unbiased sampling (Irizarry et al. 1997b; Sigurdsson et al. 2001b). Aβ deposits were analyzed under x165 magnification in the cortical ribbon extending on the superiolateral aspect of the hemisphere from the cingulate cortex to the rhinal fissure ventrally. The anatomic locations and boundaries of the cortical region analyzed were based on those defined by Franklin and Paxinos (1997). The area of the grid was 800 x 800 μm^2 and the amyloid deposits were analyzed in 18 frames per mouse (640 x 400μm^2), selected in a systematic random manner throughout the rostro-caudal axis of the brain.

Only lesions larger than 200μm^2 (i.e., larger than mean + 2 standard deviations of CA3 pyramidal neuron cross section area) were counted. The number of Aβ plaques per mm^2 and the Aβ burden was measured in each test area. The Aβ burden is defined as the percentage of area in the measurement field occupied by reaction product.

For quantitation of the amyloid burden in μMRI images, digitized tagged-image format files with a calibrated scale marker were imported into the Bioquant stereology image analysis software. The brightness of the images was altered so that the average optical density measurement for each imported image was similar. A region of interest was manually drawn on the gray matter of the cortex and on the hippocampus corresponding to the anatomical landmarks used for the histological amyloid burden quantification. Dark spots within this region of interest that had a threshold value below 110 and that were >200 μm^2 counted as "amyloid" deposits. The numerical density of lesions on μMRI was calculated by dividing the number of lesions by area of the region of interest. Since, the size of lesions on μMRI directly corresponds to the signal generated by the labeling ligands and did not correspond to the true size of the lesion as Measured by histology, we determined the numerical density of lesions rather than their total burden.

Quantification of both amyloid burden and lesions detected by μMRI was performed by an individual blinded to the genotype of the mice and the experimental protocol used. The correlation between numerical density of lesions detected by μMRI ex vivo and numerical density and burden of Aβ deposits on histological sections was analyzed using Pearsons's correlation coefficient using software package Statistica 6.1 (StatSoft Inc., Tulsa, OK).

Results

μMRI Studies

In vivo injection of purified Gd-DTPA-Aβ1-40 into the carotid artery of both 15- to 16-month-old APP transgenic mice and six-month-old APP/PS1 transgenic mice, along with 15% mannitol to transiently open the BBB, resulted in the detection of numerous dark spots, indicative of amyloid lesions, on T2 and T2*-weighted μMRI. As expected, T2*-weighted gradient echo imaging provided the most sensitiv in vivo detection method, allowing the use of thinner image slices and shorter imaging times. In contrast, dark spots similar to those seen in all AD transgenic mice were rarely observed in wild-type control mice injected and imaged using the same protocols. Blood vessels were easily identified in both Gd-DTPA-Aβ1-40 injected and control animals due to the hypointensity that probably results from deoxyhemoglobin in blood vessels. They were distinguished as long, thin structures running either completely in the plain of imaging or when cut under an angle gave them an oval shape on cross-section. They were generally smaller than lesions labeled with Gd-DTPA-Aβ1-40 deposits and less hypointense, which allowed them to be eliminated during thresholding (see quantitative analysis below). Also,vessels on cross-section rarely presented as clusters; instead their profiles were equally distributed. The few dark spots observed in μMRI of control mice were isolated, unlike the clustered patterns of spots in the AD transgenic mice, and probably corresponded to larger blood vessels.The dark spots observed in μMRI of the AD transgenic mice injected with Gd- DTPA-Aβ1-40 showed good correlation with the corresponding immunohistochemically (6E10) stained brain sections for amyloid (see Fig.2).

In vivo co-injection of MION-Aβ1-40 with 15% mannitol into the carotid arteries of 16-month-old APP transgenic mice and six-month-old APP/PS1 transgenic mice also resulted in numerous dark spots on ex vivo μMRI, which correlated well with the corresponding immunohistochemically (6E10) stained brain sections for amyloid. No dark spots were observed in the brains of wild-type mice injected with MION-Aβ1-40 plus mannitol, in 15- to 16-month-old APP transgenic mice injected with MION-Aβ1.40 without mannitol or in 15- to 16-month-old APP transgenic mice injected with MION alone (without Aβ1-40) with mannitol, although amyloid lesions were present in all of the AD transgenic mice imaged.

Correlation between μMRI and Histology

Amyloid burden, assessed by quantitative immunohistochemical analysis of tissue sections from the cortex of 15- to 16-month-old APP transgenic mice was 1.0% ± 0.68 (SD), whereas in six- month-old APP/PS1 transgenic mice the amyloid burden was 1.87% ± 0.92 (SD). These measured amyloid burdens are consistent with published data in these transgenic mice at these ages (Irizarry et al. 1997a; Takeuchi et al. 2000; Wengenack et al. 2000b).

In AD transgenic mice injected with Gd-DTPA-Aβ1-40 and mannitol, there was a statistically significant correlation between the density of lesions demonstrated by μMRI and both the density (p=0.011, r=0.871) and the total burden (p=0.023, r=0.824) of lesions detected by immunohistochemistry (see Fig. 3). Although μMRI is not detecting all amyloid lesions, the proportion of lesions detected correlates with the total number of lesions, as determined by morphometric histological studies.

The sensitivity of MION-Aβ1-40 to detect Aβ deposits was comparable to that of Gd- Aβ1-40 when corrected for the Aβ burden. The ratio of lesion density detected by μMRI on 500μm-thick slices to lesion density on 40μm histological sections was 1.3±0.1 (S.D.) for MION-Aβ1-40 and 1.1±0.3 for Gd- Aβ1-40 (S.D.). In transgenic animals injected with MION-Aβ1-40 and mannitol, the correlation between density of lesions detected by ex vivo μMRI and that on histological sections did not reach the level of statistical significance due to greater individual variability.

54   Einar M. Sigurdsson et al.

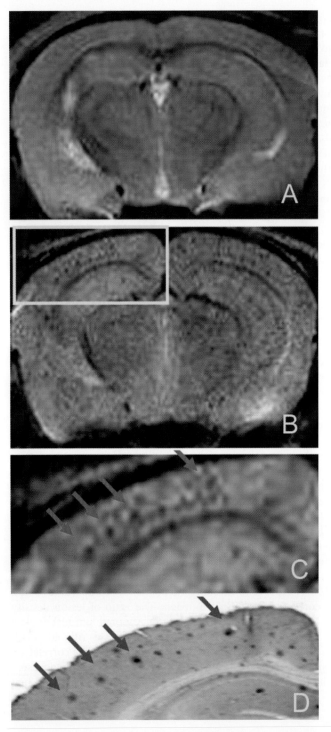

Fig. 2. Aβ plaques are detected with in vivo µMRI after injection of Gd-DTPA-Aβ1-40 with mannitol. Lesions cannot be detected without injection of ligand. **A** shows a T2 weighted µMRI of a AD model transgenic mouse, without the injection of ligand. No amyloid lesions can be detected. **B** shows a T2 weighted mMRI of the same mouse imaged in **A**, following injection of Gd-DPTA-Aβ1-40. This imaging was performed 24 hours following the scan shown in **A**. Numerous hypodense lesions are seen in the hypocampus and cortex. **C** shows a higher magnification of the area in a box shown in **B**. **D** shows a tissue section corresponding to the area shown in **C** that was immuno-reacted with anti-Aβ antibodies. The brown areas are parenchymal amyloid plaques. Several of the plaques seen in the µMRI shown in **C** and the histology in **D** co-register (see arrows).

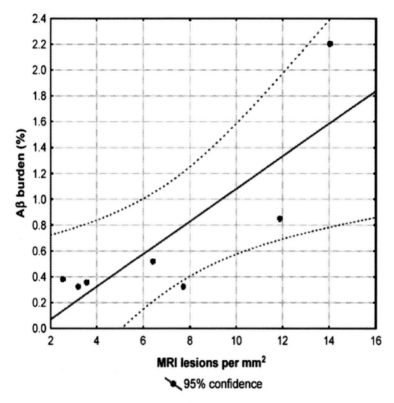

Fig. 1. A statistically significant correlation between the numerical density of lesions detected by in vivo μMRI and the total Aβ burden determined by histology (p=0.023; r=0.82).

Discussion

The presented data show that a systemic injection of Aβ1-40 peptide chelated to Gd or absorbed onto MION allows the detection of Aβ deposits by μMRI in the brains of AD transgenic mice in vivo (Wisniewski et al. 2001b; Poduslo et al. 2002; Sigurdsson et al. 2003). The imaging times are relatively short (1-2 hours) using our T2-weighted spin echo and T2*-weighted gradient echo μMRI protocols. Under these conditions, the amyloid lesions appear hypodense on MRI. By contrast, when we used T1-weighted μMRI, the detected lesions were hyperintense but required acquisition times of over 16 hours. Such a long imaging time was not feasible for in vivo studies and could only be used ex vivo. Our μMRI is specific, since mice with no amyloid lesions that were injected with Gd-DTPA-Aβ1-40 or MION-Aβ1-40 had virtually no false positive lesion. Although our technique allows for the visualization of only a portion of the total amyloid burden, this portion correlates well with the total amyloid burden found on histology (see Fig.

3). Our µMRI detection of Aβ plaques illustrates that Aβ-peptide-based amyloid ligands (Wisniewski et al. 2001b; Poduslo et al. 2002; Sigurdsson et al. 2003), with further modification to increase BBB permeability and solubility, may be useful diagnostically in AD patients in the future. Past studies have used at are not suitable for in vivo imaging. Benveniste et al. (1999) reported that they were able to detect neuritic plaques in extracted pieces of post-mortem brains from AD patients. Without using contrast agents, they found that scanning times of 20 hours were required to achieve the resolution necessary to detect Aβ plaques. However, Dhenain et al. (2002) reported that, with even better resolution, they were unable to detect Aβ plaques in brain samples from AD patients.

Our results show that the use of Aβ peptides to target Gd or MION to amyloid lesions allows for much shorter imaging times, which are more practical for in vivo neuroimaging. Our ligands preferentially lead to the detection of larger parenchymal deposits. However, despite the limitation that our ligands only visualized a portion of total lesions, the labeling clearly correlates with the total amyloid burden (see Fig. 3). Furthermore, our ligands, with thresholding, produce a very low false positive rate for lesion detection. In the AD transgenic mice and control animals used in this study, we could differentiate between controls and amyloid bearing mice with 100% sensitivity and specificity. Hence we hope that our imaging approaches will allow us and other investigators to dynamically monitor amyloid clearance while developing potential therapeutic strategies, such as ongoing studies of "amyloid vaccination" (Sigurdsson et al., 2001a, 2002).

In future studies we plan to further develop this methodology, by altering the ligand to limit potential toxicity and to increase BBB permeability, with the goal of making this method more suitable for human use. The imaging approach presented in our studies shows promise that early detection of one of the hallmarks of AD is within reach (Poduslo et al. 2002; Sigurdsson et al. 2003; Wisniewski et al. 2001b). We also believe that similar imaging approaches can be applied to other neurodegenerative disorders. AD is one of several "conformational" neurodegenerative disorders that are characterized by the deposition of a normal host protein in an abnormal, β-pleated conformation that is associated with toxicity (Wisniewski et al. 2001a, 2002). In prion diseases (such as new variant Creutzfeldt-Jakob disease) normal Prpc is converted to β-pleated Prpsc (Prusiner 2001). Ligands that specifically bind to Prpsc may allow for the early diagnosis of this group of diseases, using similar methods to what we have described for Aβ plaque detection. Studies are currently underway to develop such imaging capabilities (Sadowski et al. 2003a,b). Effective therapeutic approaches are under development for several neurodegenerative disorders. For these therapies to have a maximal effect, it is essential to have imaging methodologies that will allow an early diagnosis, prior to extensive irreversible neuronal damage.

Acknowledgments

This research was supported by the Alzheimer's Disease Association (TW) and NIH grants NS38461(DHT), GM57467 (DHT), AG15408 (TW) AG20245 (TW) and AG17617 (TW).

References

Bellin MF, Beigelman C, Precetti-Morel S (2000) Iron oxide-enhanced MR lymphography: initial experience. Eur J Radiol 34: 257–264

Benveniste H, Einstein G, Kim KR, Hulette C, Johnson GA (1999) Detection of neuritic plaques in Alzheimer's disease by magnetic resonance microscopy. Proc Natl Acad Sci USA 96: 14079–14084

Chi OZ, Chang Q, Wang G, Weiss HR (1997) Effects of nitric oxide on blood-brain barrier disruption caused by intracarotid injection of hyperosmolar mannitol in rats. Anesth Analg 84: 370–375

Cosolo WC, Martinello P, Louis WJ, Chrisophidis N (1989) Blood-brain barrier disruption using mannitol: time course and electron microscopy studies. Am J Physiol 256: R443–R447

Dhenain M, Privat N, Duyckaerts C, Jacobs RE (2002) Senile plaques do not induce susceptibility effects in T2* weighted MR microscopic images. NMR Biomed 15: 197–203

Enochs WS, Harsh G, Hochberg F, Weissleder R (1999) Improved delineation of human brain tumors on MR images using a long-circulating, superparamagnetic iron oxide agent. J Magn Reson Imag 9: 228–232

Franklin KBJ, Paxinos G (1997) The mouse brain in stereotaxic coordinates. London, Academic Press.

Harisinghani MG, Saini S, Slater GJ, Schnall MD, Rifkin MD (1997) MR imaging of pelvic lymph nodes in primary pelvic carcinoma with ultrasmall superparamagnetic iron oxide (Combidex): preliminary observations. J Magn Reson Imag 7: 161–163

Harisinghani MG, Saini S, Weissleder R, Hahn PF, Yantiss RK, Tempany C, Wood BJ, Mueller PR (1999) MR lymphangiography using ultrasmall superparamagnetic iron oxide in patients with primary abdominal and pelvic malignancies: radiographic-pathologic correlation. AJRL Am J Roentgenol 172: 1347–1351

Harisinghani MG, Saini S, Weissleder R, Rubin D, deLange E, Harms S, Weinreb J, Small W, Sukerkar A, Brown JJ, Zelch J, Lucas M, Morris M, Hahn PF (2001) Splenic imaging with ultrasmall superparamagnetic iron oxide ferumoxtran-10 (AMI-7227): preliminary observations. J Comp Assist Tomog 25: 770–776

Holcomb L, Gordon MN, McGowan E, Yu X, Benkovic S, Jantzen P, Saad WK, Mueller R, Morgan D, Sanders S, Zehr C, O'Campo K, Hardy J, Prada CM, Eckman C, Younkin S, Hsiao K, Duff K (1998) Accelerated Alzheimer-type phenotype in transgenic mice carrying both mutant amyloid precursor protein and presenilin 1 transgenes. Nature Med 4: 97–100

Hsiao KK, Chapman P, Nilsen S, Eckman C, Harigaya Y, Younkin S, Yang F, Cole G (1996) Correlative memory deficits, Aβ elevation and amyloid plaques in transgenic mice. Science 274: 99–102

Irizarry MC, McNamara M, Fedorchak K, Hsiao K, Hyman BT (1997a) APPSw transgenic mice develop age-related Aβ deposits and neuropil abnormalities, but no neuronal loss in CA1. J Neuropathol Exp Neurol 56: 965–973

Irizarry MC, Soriano F, McNamara M, Page KJ, Schenk D, Games D, Hyman BT (1997b) Aβ deposition is associated with neuropil changes, but not with overt neuronal loss in the human amyloid precursor protein V717F (PDAPP) transgenic mouse. J Neurosci 17: 7053–7059

Janus C, Pearson J, McLaurin J, Mathews PM, Jiang Y, Schmidt SD, Chishti MA, Horne P, Heslin D, French J, Mount HT, Nixon RA, Mercken M, BergeronC, Fraser PE, George-Hyslop P, Westaway D (2000) Aβ peptide immunization reduces behavioural impairment and plaques in a model of Alzheimer's disease. Nature 408: 979–982

Jarrett JT, Lansbury PT, Jr (1993) Seeding "one-dimensional crystallization" of amyloid: a pathogenic mechanism in Alzheimer's disease and scrapie? Cell 73: 1055-1058

Kim KS, Wen GY, Bancher C, Chen CMJ, Sapienza V, Hong H, Wisniewski HM (1990) Detection and quantification of amyloid β-peptide with 2 monoclonal antibodies. Neurosci Res Commun 7: 113–122

Lee HJ, Zhang Y, Zhu C, Duff K, Partridge WM (2002) Imaging brain amyloid of Alzheimer disease in vivo in transgenic mice with an Aβ peptide radiopharmaceutical. J Cereb Blood Flow Metab 22: 223–231

Mackic JB, Bading J, Ghiso J, Walker L, Wisniewski T, Frangione B, Zlokovic B (2002) Transport across the blood-brain barrier and differential cerebrovascular sequestration of circulating Alzheimer's amyloid-β peptide in aged Rhesus versus aged Squirrel monkeys. Vasc Pharmacol 38:303–313

Maggio JE, Stimson ER, Ghilardi JR, Allen CJ, Dahl CE, Whitcomb DC, Vigna SR, Vinters HV, Labenski ME, Mantyh PW (1992) Reversible in vitro growth of Alzheimer disease beta-amyloid plaques by deposition of labeled amyloid peptide. Proc Natl Acad of Sci USA 89: 5462–5466

Marshall JR, Stimson ER, Ghilardi JR, Vinters HV, Mantyh PW, Maggio JE (2002) Noninvasive imaging of peripherally injected Alzheimer's disease type synthetic Aβ amyloid in vivo. Bioconjugate Chem 13: 276–284

Moore A, Weissleder R, Bogdanov A (1997) Uptake of dextran-coated monocyrstalline iron oxide in tumor cells and macrophages. J Magnet Reson Imag 7: 1140–1145

Morgan D, Diamond, DM, Gottschall PE, Ugen KE, Dickey C, Hardy J, Duff K, Jantzen P, DiCarlo G, Wilcock D, Connor K, Hatcher J, HopeC, Gordon M, Arendash GW (2001) Aβ peptide vaccination prevents memory loss in an animal model of Alzheimer's disease. Nature 408: 982–985

Morri JC (1999) Is Alzheimer's disease inevitable with age? Lessons from clinicopathologic studies of healthy aging and very mild Alzheimer's disease.J Clin Invest 104: 1171-1173

Nguyen BC, Stanford W, Thompson BH, Rossi NP, Kernstine KH, Kern JA, Robinson RA, Amorosa JK, Mammone JF, Outwater EK (1999) Multicenter clinical trial of ultrasmall superparamagnetic iron oxide in the evaluation of mediastinal lymph nodes in patients with primary lung carcinoma. J Magnet Res Imag 10: 468–473

Poduslo JF, Wengenack TM, Curran GL, Wisniewski T, Sigurdsson EM, Macura SI, Borowski BJ, Jack CR (2002) Molecular contrast enhanced magnetic resonance imaging of Alzheimer's amyloid plaques. Neurobiol Dis 11: 315–329

Price JL, Morris JC (1999) Tangles and plaques in nondemented aging and «preclinical» Alzheimer's disease. Ann Neurol 45: 358–368

Prusiner SB (2001) Neurodegenerative diseases and prions. New Engl J Med 344: 1516–1526

Sadowski M, Tang CY, Aguilanldo JG, Carp RI, Wadghiri YZ, Turnbull D, Wisniewski T (2003a) MRI approaches for the detection of prion disease pathology. Am Acad Neurol Meeting

Sadowski M, Tang CY, Aguilanldo JG, Carp RI, Wisniewski T (2003b) In vivo Micro-MRI signal changes in scrapie infected mice. Neurosci Lett, 345:1-4

Schenk D, Barbour R, Dunn W, Gordon G, Grajeda H, Guido T, Hu K, Huang J, Johnson-Wood K, Khan K, Kholodenko D, Lee M, Liao Z, Lieberburg I, Motter R, Mutter L, Soriano F, Shopp G, Vasquez N, Vandevert C, Walker S, Wogulis M, Yednock T, Games D, Seubert P (1999) Immunization with amyloid-β attenuates Alzheimer disease-like pathology in the PDAPP mice. Nature 400: 173–177

Shen T, Weissleder R, Papisov M, Bogdanov A, Brady TJ (1993) Moncrystalline iron oxide nanocompounds (MION): Physiochemical properties. Magn Res Med 29: 599–604

Siegal T, Rubinstein R, Bokstein F, Schwartz A, Lossos A, Shalom E, Chisin R, Gomori JM (2000) In vivo assessment of the window of barrier opening after osmotic blood-brain barrier disruption in humans. J Neurosurg 92: 599–605

Sigurdsson EM, Scholtzova H, Mehta P, Frangione B, Wisniewski T (2001a) Immunization with a non-toxic/non-fibrillar amyloid-β homologous peptide reduces Alzheimer's disease associated pathology in transgenic mice. Am J Pathol 159: 439–447

Sigurdsson EM, Scholtzova H, Mehta P, Frangione B, Wisniewski T (2001b) Immunization with a nontoxic/nonfibrillar amyloid-β homologous peptide reduces Alzheimer's disease associated pathology in transgenic mice. Am J Pathol 159: 439–447

Sigurdsson EM, Brown DR, Daniels M, Kascsak RJ, Kascsak R, Carp RI, Meeker HC, Frangione B, Wisniewski T (2002) Vaccination delays the onset of prion disease in mice. Am J Pathol 161: 13–17

Sigurdsson EM, Z aim Wadghiri Y, Sadowski M, Tang CY, Aguilanldo JG, Elliot JI, Li Y, Pappolla MA, Duff K, Turnbull D, Wisniewski T (2003) Detection of Alzheimer's amyloid lesions in transgenic mice by magnetic resonance imaging. Magn Res Med, 50:293–302

Skovronsky DM, Zhang B, Mei-Ping K, Kung HF, Trojanowski JQ, Lee VMY (2000) In vivo detection of amyloid plaques in a mouse model of Alzheimer's disease. Proc Natl Acad Sci USA 97: 7609–7614

Takeuchi A, Irizarry MC, Duff K, Saido T, Hsiao Ashe K, Hasegawa H, Mann DM, Hyman BT, Iwatsubo T (2000) Age-related amyloid β deposition in transgenic mice overexpressing both Alzheimer mutant presenilin 1 and amyloid β precursor protein swedish mutant is not associated with global neuronal loss. Am J Pathol 157: 331–339

Weissleder R, Mahmood U, Bhorade R, Benveniste H, Chiocca EA, Basilion JP (2000). In vivo magnetic resonance imaging of transgene expression. Nature Med 6: 351–354

Wengenack TM, Curran GL, Poduslo JF (2000a) Targeting Alzheimer amyloid plaques in vivo. Nature Biotech 18: 868–872

Wengenack TM, Whelan S, Curran GL, Duff KE, Poduslo JF (2000b) Quantitative histological analysis of amyloid deposition in Alzheimer's double transgenic mouse brain. Neuroscience 101: 939–944

Wisniewski T, Sigurdsson EM, Aucouturier P, Frangione B (2001a) Conformation as a therapeuctic target in the prionoses and other neurodegenerative conditions. In: Baker HF (ed) Molecular and cellular pathology in prion disease. Totowa, New Jersey, Humana Press, pp. 223–236

Wisniewski T, Wadghiri YZ, Elliot JI, Pappolla M, Duff K, Turnbull D, Sigurdsson EM (2001b) Detection of Alzheimer's amyloid by magnetic resonance imaging. Soc Neurosci Abst 27:1217

Wisniewski T, Brown DR, Sigurdsson EM (2002) Therapeutics in Alzheimer's and prion diseases. Biochem Soc Transact 30: 574–578

Xu S, Jordan EK, Brocke S, Bulte JWM, Quigley L, Tresser N, Ostuni JL, Yang Y, McFarland HF, Frank JA (1998) Study of relapsing remitting experimental allergic encephalomyelitis SJL mouse model: using MION-46L enhancing in vivo MRI: early histopathological correlation. J Neurosci Res 52: 549–558

Measuring Progression in Alzheimer's Disease using Serial MRI: 4D MRI

N.C. Fox[1], J.M. Schott[1], and *R.I. Scahill[1]*

Summary

In this chapter, we discuss the utility of magnetic resonance imaging (MRI) in the diagnosis and assessment of progression in Alzheimer's disease (AD). Whilst MRI has been typically used to exclude alternative causes of dementia, it is increasingly used to aid a positive diagnosis. Serial imaging allows progression to be demonstrated, and novel techniques, which use accurate scan matching, allow direct comparison and calculation of both global and regional change. These measures may be useful both as outcome measures in clinical trials and for early diagnosis.

Introduction

A defining feature of the neurodegenerative disorders is their inexorable progression. AD is associated with an insidious onset of episodic memory difficulties, followed by an accrual of ever wider cognitive deficits and behavioural problems. These deficits ultimately lead to the breakdown of all higher cognitive functions, loss of independent living and a decreased life span. In AD, the pathological substrate for this gradual functional decline is neuronal and synaptic loss associated with an accumulation of amyloid plaques and neurofibrillary tangles within the brain (Braak and Braak, 1991). Typically this histopathological progression follows a region-specific sequence, with tangles appearing first in entorhinal cortex and then hippocampus, before progressing to involve the association cortices (Braak and Braak, 1991). Over the last few decades our understanding of this inexorable progression has increased dramatically; to date, however, no therapies have been developed to halt this process. Whilst symptomatic therapies that may provide some transient improvement in cognitive functioning are now available (Corey Bloom et al. 1998; Rogers et al. 1998), the next and crucial challenge is to develop drugs that will slow disease progression. With several potential disease-modifying agents in development, this prospect is perhaps within reach. With these advances come new challenges for imaging research in AD.

---

[1] Institute of Neurology, Queen Square, London,WC1N 3BG, U.K

Hyman et al.
The Living Brain and Alzheimer's
©Springer-Verlag Berlin Heidelberg

Historically, imaging in AD has largely been used to exclude alternative causes of cognitive decline that might be potentially treatable. However, recent advances in image resolution and the increasing range of acquisition sequences available have provided the opportunity for MRI to play a more significant role in the diagnosis of dementia. For example, a volumetric 3-dimensional MRI scan can be acquired in under 10 minutes and provides detail of the structure of the brain down to a resolution of 1mm (Fox et al. 2001b). As our understanding of the neuroradiological features of AD has improved, so too has our ability to use MRI to aid in the positive diagnosis of the disease (Scheltens et al. 2002). In particular, improved acquisition sequences have increased our ability to determine the presence and degree of cerebrovascular disease (Erkinjuntti et al. 1999).

Clinical Trial Design

Over the last few years, there has been increasing interest in using MR imaging in therapeutic trials designed to assess progression of the disease. To date, clinical trials assessing therapeutic agents in AD have relied on neuropsychological and functional scores, such as the Alzheimer Disease Assessment Scale-cognitive (ADAS-cog; (Rosen et al. 1984)), as outcome measures. Such measures have poor sensitivity to change because of a lack of reproducibility; they are also subject to floor and ceiling effects and practice effects and may be influenced by anxiety. These problems may be compounded by the fact that AD appears to be heterogeneous in terms of clinical or cognitive progression. It follows that large trials are required to show effects using traditional measures. Furthermore, differentiating symptomatic effects from true, disease-slowing benefit is more difficult still and requires logistically and ethically complicated trial designs involving staggered start or withdrawal or crossover studies (Leber, 1996). The costs involved in undertaking such trials are therefore considerable, and the stakes are high. Taking an ineffective therapy forward into clinical trials may lead to patients being exposed to unnecessary risks while significant resources are wasted; missing a potentially useful therapy will inevitably result in huge losses to patients and to society at large. It would be extremely valuable to be able to reduce the size and/or duration of these trials without sacrificing power to detect a real effect on disease progression. There are several ways in which MRI may help with these issues.

Cross-sectional imaging: aiding accurate diagnosis

A truly disease-modifying agent is likely to have a pathology-specific mechanism of action. The inclusion of patients with non-AD pathology weakens a trial of any such agent, and consequently there is a growing need for early and accurate diagnosis. Whilst no cross-sectional imaging techniques are yet able definitively to diagnose AD, an MRI scan showing symmetrical hippocampal atrophy and a relative absence of ischaemic changes has been shown to add significant positive predictive value to the clinical diagnosis (Scheltens et al. 2002). Furthermore, these features increase the probability of a patient with the earliest symptoms of memory impairment (mild cognitive impairment – MCI) progressing to a diagnosis of AD (Jack et al. 1999). This provides the potential to include patients with very early disease in treatment studies; it is likely that this group who have yet to develop significant impairment will derive most benefit from disease-modifying agents.

Longitudinal MRI: Measuring Progression

MRI measures of cerebral atrophy are increasingly being considered as markers of progression. Progression markers are important in understanding the disease process and in providing prognostic information to patients and their carers. Crucially, they may also provide cost-effective ways of identifying therapies that slow disease as opposed to only providing symptomatic benefit.

Ideally, a surrogate marker of disease progression should relate directly to the nature and extent of the underlying pathology: in the case of AD, neuronal loss, amyloid and abnormal tau deposition in brain tissue. Such measures are currently under investigation (Bacskai et al. 2002), but none is yet available *in vivo*. An inevitable downstream event, which is nevertheless central to pathological progression in AD, is cerebral atrophy. High resolution volumetric MRI scans, when acquired serially from the same patient over a period of time, can be used to provide measurement of macroscopic cerebral loss. This cerebral atrophy can act as an *in vivo* marker of structural progression. Atrophy can be assessed repeatedly and non-invasively and may provide an unbiased marker of progression; if a treatment were to be truly disease-modifying, it would be expected to slow neuronal destruction and thereby slow the rate of atrophy.

Longitudinal MR Imaging: Regional Measures

Conventional MR measures of cerebral atrophy have assessed regions that are known to be affected early and prominently in AD, e.g., the entorhinal cortex and hippocampus. Such measures have traditionally required manual outlining of a region of interest. The labour-intensive nature of this technique means that only a limited number of structures can feasibly be measured and *a priori* decisions need to be made regarding which areas are to be assessed. Furthermore, such measures rely on subjective boundary placement and are subject to reproducibility problems. Nonetheless, several studies have shown hippocampal volumes to be reduced by around 25% by the time a patient with AD is mildly affected (Jack et al. 1997; Lehericy et al. 1994). Longitudinal studies have shown that rates of entorhinal cortex and hippocampal atrophy are significantly increased in AD (3–6%/year) compared to matched controls (1–2%/y; (Jack et al. 1998; Scahill et al. 2003; Schott et al. 2003a)). However, there is a wide range of atrophy rates both within and between these studies; whilst some of this variability might be related to true disease heterogeneity, some may also reflect measurement error. Typical scan-rescan measurement errors are around 3–5% for the hippocampus (Schott et al. 2003a) – importantly, this is of the same order of magnitude as the changes one is trying to measure. Recent work has focussed on the development of automated template-based regional segmentation techniques, which have the potential to re-duce operator time and improve reproducibility greatly (Andreasen et al. 1996; Collins et al. 1996; Csernansky et al. 1998). However, these methods generally rely on landmark identification, and are currently limited by large inter-subject vari-ability, particularly in a disease as heterogeneous as AD.

Longitudinal MR Imaging: Global Atrophy Measures

Whilst medial temporal lobe volume losses may be evident at the earliest stages of AD, by the time of diagnosis it is clear that generalised cerebral loss and ven-tricular enlargement are also proceeding rapidly (DeCarli et al. 1992; Schott et al. 2003a). Thus measures of global atrophy are also plausible measures of disease progression. Whilst the annualized percentage changes may be smaller than for individual structures such as the hippocampus, global changes can be measured with greater precision and may prove to be more efficient and more robust. In ad-dition, by assessing the whole brain, *a priori* judgements about which structures should be assessed are avoided, and thus change occurring in less predictable areas of the brain will not be discounted.

To measure the rate of global cerebral atrophy within an individual, it is neces-sary to compare two or more brain scans, acquired with the same MRI parameters over a known time interval. By subtracting the second brain image from the first, the difference, equating to the volume of brain loss, can be assessed. This mea-sure can be converted to an annual global brain atrophy rate by correcting for the inter-scan interval. A major obstacle to this approach is that it is extremely diffi-cult to scan an individual in exactly the same position and orientation twice. This problem has been overcome by the development of computer algorithms capable of accurately aligning a 3D follow-up scan onto the baseline. There are numerous methods that are now available to perform this positional matching (Collins et al. 1994; Woods et al. 1998); one such technique is linear, or 9 degrees of freedom, registration (Freeborough et al. 1996).

Accurate Scan Matching: Linear (9 Degrees of Freedom) Registration

This process involves calculating the translations (along 3 axes), rotations (around 3 axes) and linear scalings (in 3 dimensions) required to match the brain volumes one on top of the other. This technique is driven by minimizing the difference in the voxel signal intensity (i.e., matching grey voxels to grey, white to white, etc.) between the two scans, and relies on the complexity of the brain to ensure there is only one perfect match. Using this technique, serial scans can be matched very precisely to a sub-voxel level, with mean point matching of the order of 0.2 to 0.4 mm over the whole brain (Freeborough et al. 1996; Hajnal et al. 1995). Once reg-istered, differences may be appreciated by comparing the baseline and registered image, subtracting the images from one another, or instructing the computer to colour voxels changing intensity by more than a given percentage (Fig. 1). Fur-thermore, the accuracy of regional atrophy measures calculated from manual

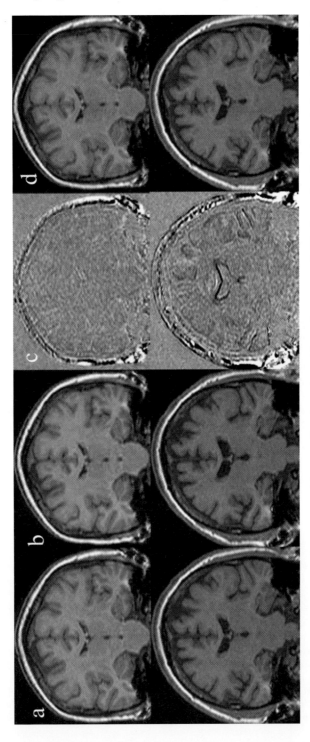

Fig. 1. MR images are shown from a healthy control (top panel) and a patient with AD (bottom panel). The first, or baseline, image is shown in a, with the registered repeat, approximately a year later, in b. Excellent positional matching is seen in both; expansion of the ventricles reflecting excess global atrophy is evident in the patient with AD. This is confirmed in the difference image (c), and is shown in panel d, where significant tissue loss is highlighted in red.

outlining may be improved, if such measurements are made on registered pairs of images.

Automated Calculation of Atrophy:
The Brain Boundary Shift Integral

As with regional atrophy measures, global brain atrophy can be calculated by manually outlining the whole brain volume on two serial scans and calculating the change between them. Whilst performing these measurements on registered images improves accuracy, this process is still operator-intensive and open to problems of bias and measurement error. A measure of global brain atrophy, the brain boundary shift integral (BBSI) can be calculated directly from the difference images (Freeborough and Fox, 1997). This technique relies on measuring and summing the voxel shift that occurs at the brain/cerebrospinal fluid interface and allows quantification of volume changes that have occurred in the interval between the scans (Fig. 2). Global atrophy rates may be measured in this way directly, semi-automatically and with high precision (0.2% of whole brain volume; (Freeborough and Fox, 1997)), and atrophy rates derived using this technique have been shown to correlate with clinical decline (Fox et al. 1999a).

Using registration and the BBSI technique to measure atrophy rates in a retrospective study of clinically diagnosed patients scanned twice, one year apart, it was shown that the annualised mean (standard deviation) rate of brain atrophy in AD is 2.4% (1.1), which compares to 0.4% (0.4) in age-matched controls (Fox et al. 2000). Using these rates, it is possible to derive estimates of sample sizes that would be required in each arm of a placebo-controlled study investigating the effects of a novel therapy on disease progression. Allowing for 10% of scans to be unusable, and 10% of patients dropping out (both reasonable assumptions in a clinical trial), it was estimated that 207 subjects per treatment arm would pro-

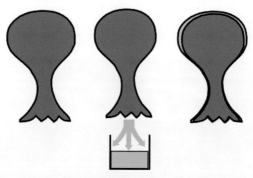

Fig. 2 Cartoon depicting the principles of the BBSI. If a balloon filled with water (left) has some of the water released (center), the balloon will shrink at its edges (right). The sum of the total distances the balloon edges move by will equate to the volume of water lost. In the case of the brain, cerebral atrophy will result in an increase in the size of cerebrospinal fluid (CSF) spaces. The BBSI measures the shift in the brain/CSF boundary across the whole brain volume, which provides a direct, automated measure of brain volume loss.

vide 90% power at a 5% level to detect a 20% reduction in atrophy rate (Fox et al. 2000). In a prospective study of aged patients with AD and appropriate controls scanned over one year, the rates of brain atrophy were remarkably similar. Thus the annualized atrophy rate was 2.19% (0.82) in AD patients and 0.53% (0.58) in controls, leading to estimated sample sizes of 144 per treatment arm (Schott et al. 2003c). These sample size estimates are significantly lower than those required if clinical scales (e.g., ADAS-Cog) are used and are similar to estimations based on manual hippocampal measures (Jack et al. 2003). One assumption of these power calculations (that appears reasonable) is that the most one could expect from a therapeutic agent would be to slow atrophy rates to the levels seen in controls. Global atrophy rates in controls are age-related (Scahill et al. 2003), and it is therefore important that subgroups within studies are well matched for age.

Several studies of individuals at risk of familial AD have shown that rates of atrophy accelerate very gradually and are already significantly raised two to three years prior to symptom declaration (Fox et al. 1999b; Schott et al. 2003a). As atrophy rates are similar in patients with sporadic and familial AD, this finding leads to several important conclusions. First, this technique may be useful in treatment trials assessing the effects of drugs on the very earliest stages of the disease, at which time disease modification would be most likely to have greatest effect. Second, the slow rate of acceleration in AD means that, over periods of one to two years, whole brain volume losses can be considered to be linear. This finding has important implications for study design. If, as seems the case, within-subject variability in rates of atrophy is lower than the between-subject variability, then there may be significant advantages in running studies that are more focussed on measuring changes in individual rates of atrophy. This leads the way to novel trial design, with, for example, patients having three or more scans during the study, with a run-in period before randomisation to a treatment or placebo arm. Despite concerns that patients with AD are unable to tolerate serial MRI scans, it has recently been shown that, with care, patients are remarkably tolerant of serial imaging. In a one-year prospective study of 28 patients with mild to moderate AD, which involved ten MRI scans at seven different time-points, the patient drop-out rate was under 10% (Schott et al. 2003c). Thus multiple time-point imaging is feasible in AD and may improve the power of these registration-based techniques to identify disease-modifying effects.

Non-linear Registration

The linear registration technique described above treats the brain as a rigid body. Whilst adequate for measuring global brain losses, these methods are unable to detect localised changes occurring within the brain, merely highlighting change at the brain/CSF boundaries (Fig. 1). There are inevitable structural changes that occur during the process of neurodegeneration, and, in AD, it is known that different brain regions are the focus of the pathological process at different stages of the disease (Braak and Braak, 1991). The ability to map these changes would provide valuable information about the ongoing patterns of regional atrophy, which in turn might help both with differentiating diseases on the basis of their specific pattern of atrophy and monitoring their progression. One way to detect such changes is to match an individual's serial imaging using non-linear methods.

Detecting changes in individuals

The term "fluid registration" (Christensen et al. 1996) has been used to describe a subset of non-linear warping techniques based on the physical model of a compressible viscous fluid. Novel image analysis methods based on this model that allow localised/regional atrophy to be visualized and calculated from serial MRI scans have been developed (Crum et al. 2001; Freeborough and Fox, 1998). This methodology requires an initial rigid body registration (as described above) to match the scans exactly and a second, non-linear "fluid" registration to determine contraction or expansion on a voxel-by voxel basis. Voxel compression maps are then generated that show the distribution of these changes over the whole brain, highlighting areas undergoing contraction or expansion. In individuals with AD, this technique has demonstrated presymptomatic atrophy focussed on medial

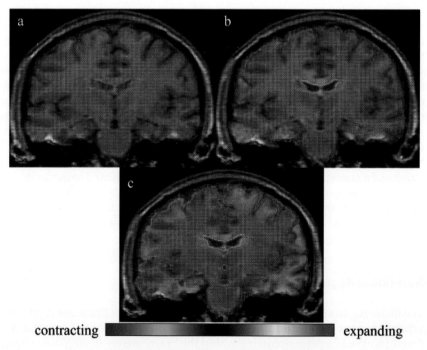

contracting ▬▬▬▬▬▬▬▬▬▬▬▬▬▬▬▬▬ expanding

Fig. 3. Voxel compression maps (VCM) derived from fluid-registration of serial MRI scans are shown in a patient with familial AD. Image **a** shows the changes occurring over a period prior to the onset of symptoms. Early hippocampal atrophy and mild ventricular enlargement are shown. Image **b** shows the same individual's serial scan spanning the time he/she became symptomatic. Increasing temporal lobe atrophy and ventricular expansion are seen. The patient subsequently fulfilled clinical criteria for the diagnosis of AD. Image **c** shows the VCM covering

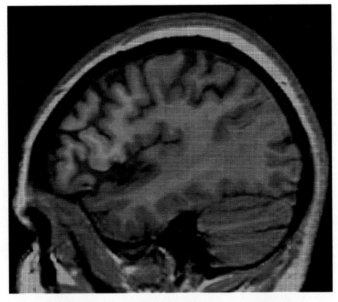

contracting ▬▬▬▬▬▬▬▬▬▬▬▬▬▬▬ expanding

Fig. 4. Serial sagittal MRI with voxel compression mapping overlay is shown from a patient with presymptomatic familial frontotemporal lobar degeneration over the time period when symptoms (speech production difficulties) first appeared. The figure shows focal anterolateral left frontal lobe atrophy centred around Broca's area.

temporal lobe structures and the cingulate gyrus, progressing to more significant temporal and parietal cortical losses as the disease advances (Fox et al. 2001a). In familial frontotemporal lobar degeneration, fluid registration has been applied to localise presymptomatic atrophy; the location of the very focal accelerating atrophy in one such case was centred around Broca's area and preceded the earliest signs of speech production difficulties by over a year (Janssen et al. 2002). This technique also allows the *in vivo* delineation of specific focal patterns of other neurodegenerative diseases, such as multiple system atrophy (Schott et al. 2003b). As different neurodegenerative diseases are associated with different, specific patterns of regional atrophy, fluid registration of serial MRI may be a powerful diagnostic tool in individual cases. Furthermore, as regional atrophy has been shown to precede the onset of symptoms, this technique may also aid very early diagnosis, when specific treatment targeted to the pathology in question is likely to have maximum benefits.

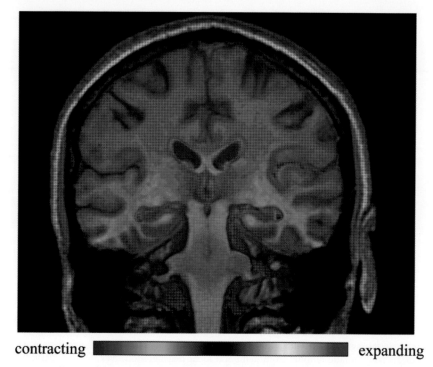

contracting ▮▮▮▮▮▮▮▮▮▮▮▮▮▮▮▮▮▮▮▮▮▮▮ expanding

Fig. 5. A sagittal MRI image with voxel compression mapping overlay from a patient with pathologically confirmed multiple system atrophy is illustrated. Greatest rates of atrophy are demonstrated in the pons and middle cerebellar peduncles and the immediately adjacent midbrain and medulla. These findings matched those found at post-mortem.

Allowing Propagation of Regions

Another potentially powerful use of fluid registration is its ability to match regions defined on a baseline scan to the same region on a subsequent scan. Using this methodology, it has been demonstrated that a hippocampus manually outlined on a baseline scan can be propagated onto a registered serial scan, and the volume of this second hippocampus can be accurately and automatically derived (Crum et al. 2001). This advance has the potential both to minimize operator error inherent in manual outlining and to reduce radically operator time. In due course, it may be possible to apply predefined brain templates, on which multiple brain regions have been defined, and possible for the fluid-registration algorithm to automatically outline and calculate the volumes of these regions on one or more serial scans. Atrophy rates from one or more of these regions could be used, depending on the nature of the disease under investigation and its stage, as trial outcome measures.

Non-linear registration: group studies

The non-linear techniques described above allow the identification of sites undergoing regional atrophy in individuals. The heterogeneous nature of AD means that there may be significant variation in the patterns of regional atrophy occurring between individuals with AD. To be a useful tool for drug studies, and to provide an important insight into the natural history of the neurodegenerative diseases, it is important to determine those brain regions consistently undergoing regional change within groups of individuals.

Fluid registration can be used to generate images consisting of approximately one million three-dimensional voxels, each containing a (Jacobian) value representing the degree of expansion or contraction required to match the second scan to the first (Freeborough and Fox, 1998). These values can be interrogated using robust statistical methods, such as those contained within the statistical parametric mapping (SPM) package (Friston et al. 1995). Prior to statistical analysis, it is essential that all scans be in the same spatial framework, so that any given voxel corresponds to exactly the same anatomical site in different individuals. SPM may then be employed to assess significant differences in either contraction or expansion on a voxel-by-voxel basis, comparing controls and groups of subjects. This methodology has been used to demonstrate altering patterns of atrophy during the progression of AD (Scahill et al. 2002). Groups of presymptomatic individuals destined to develop familial AD and patients with mild and moderate disease were compared to age-matched controls. Presymptomatic patients showed significantly increased rates of atrophy only in the hippocampus, precuneus and cingulate gyrus. By the time the disease was established but mild, increasing areas undergoing significant atrophy were seen; the disease focus had spread more laterally within the temporal lobes, and there was increasing involvement of the cingulate and association cortices. By the time the disease was moderately advanced, the highest rates of atrophy were seen in the lateral temporal lobes and cingulate, and there was widespread parietal and increasing frontal lobe atrophy (Scahill et al. 2002). These changes mirror the known histopathological progression of the disease and demonstrate the altering foci of atrophy during the progression of AD. This methodology may be a useful means of assessing areas undergoing consistent regional atrophy within groups, and it has the potential to be an unbiased method of assessing the impact of disease-modifying drugs, particularly if they were to have region-specific effects.

Conclusions

Cross-sectional MRI provides a detailed and accurate three-dimensional view of the brain. These images can aid in diagnosis, but the large inter-individual variation that exists within the population results in a large overlap between subject groups. Change over time, in the form of progressive cerebral loss, is common to all degenerative diseases. Serial MRI with accurate image registration now allows global and regional change to be visualised and quantified. Drugs that halt

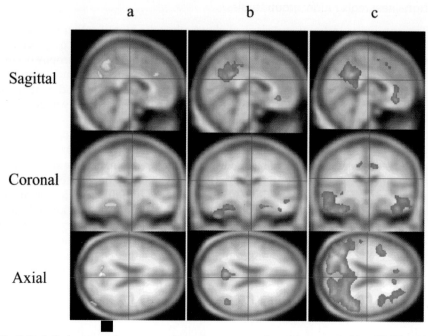

Fig. 6. Statistical parametric maps are shown from groups of presymptomatic (**a**), mild (**b**), and moderately affected (**c**) patients with AD, compared with groups of age-matched controls. Areas undergoing consistent, significantly increased rates of regional atrophy are highlighted by the colour overlay. The areas undergoing maximally increased rates of regional atrophy alter during the progression of the disease. Initially, atrophy is focussed on the hippocampi and cingulate gyri; as the disease advances, there is a shift from medial to lateral temporal lobe atrophy, with increasing parietal and frontal lobe atrophy.

the inexorable progression of this devastating disease are urgently needed; these techniques may prove to be invaluable tools in determining their efficacy.

References

Andreasen NC, Rajarethinam R, Cizadlo T, Arndt S, Swayze VW, Flashman LA, O'Leary DS, Ehrhardt JC, Yuh WT (1996) Automatic atlas-based volume estimation of human brain regions from MR images. J Comput Assist Tomogr 20:98–106

Bacskai BJ, Klunk WE, Mathis CA, Hyman BT (2002) Imaging amyloid-beta deposits in vivo. J Cereb Blood Flow Metab 22:1035–1041

Braak H, Braak E (1991) Neuropathological staging of Alzheimer-related changes. Acta Neuropathol 82:239–259

Christensen GE, Rabbitt RD, Miller MI (1996) Deformable templates using large deformation kinematics. IEEE Trans Image Proc 5:1435–1447

Collins DL, Neelin P, Peters TM, Evans AC (1994) Automatic 3D intersubject registration of MR volumetric data in standardized Talairach space. J Comput Assist Tomogr 18:192–205

Collins DL, Holmes CJ, Peters TM, Evans AC (1996) Automatic 3-D model-based neuroanatomical segmentation. Human Brain Mapp 3:190–208

Corey Bloom J, Anand R, Veach J (1998) A randomized trial evaluating the efficacy and safety of ENA 713 (rivastigmine tartrate), a new acetylcholinesterase inhibitor, in patients with mild to moderately severe Alzheimer's disease. Int J Geriat Psychopharm 1:55-65

Crum WR, Scahill RI, Fox NC (2001) Automated hippocampal segmentation by regional fluid registration of serial MRI: validation and application in Alzheimer's disease. Neuroimage 13:847–855

Csernansky JG, Joshi S, Wang L, Haller JW, Gado M, Miller JP, Grenander U, Miller MI. (1998) Hippocampal morphometry in schizophrenia by high dimensional brain mapping. Proc Natl Acad Sci (USA) 95:11406–11411

DeCarli C, Haxby JV, Gillette JA, Teichberg D, Rapoport SI, Schapiro MB (1992) Longitudinal changes in lateral ventricular volume in patients with dementia of the Alzheimer type. Neurology 42:2029–2036

Erkinjuntti T, Bowler JV, DeCarli CS, Fazekas F, Inzitari D, O'Brien JT, Pantoni L, Rockwood K, Scheltens P, Wahlund LO, Desmond DW (1999) Imaging of static brain lesions in vascular dementia: implications for clinical trials. Alzheimer Dis Assoc Disord 3:S81–90

Fox NC, Scahill RI, Crum WR, Rossor MN (1999a) Correlation between rates of brain atrophy and cognitive decline in AD. Neurology 52:1687–1689

Fox NC, Warrington EK, Rossor MN (1999b) Serial magnetic resonance imaging of cerebral atrophy in preclinical Alzheimer's disease. Lancet 353:2125

Fox NC, Cousens S, Scahill R, Harvey RJ, Rossor MN (2000) Using serial registered brain magnetic resonance imaging to measure disease progression in Alzheimer disease: power calculations and estimates of sample size to detect treatment effects. Arch Neurol 57:339–344

Fox NC, Crum WR, Scahill RI, Stevens JM, Janssen JC, Rossor MN (2001a) Imaging of onset and progression of Alzheimer's disease with voxel-compression mapping of serial magnetic resonance images. Lancet 358:201–205

Fox NC, Scahill RI, Hogh P, Rossor MN (2001b) Alzheimer's disease and neuroimaging. In: Dawbarn D, Allen S.J (eds) Neurobiology of Alzheimer's disease. Second edition. Oxford, Oxford University Press, pp 312–337

Freeborough PA, Fox NC (1997) The boundary shift integral: an accurate and robust measure of cerebral volume changes from registered repeat MRI. IEEE Trans Med Imaging 16:623–629

Freeborough PA, Fox NC (1998) Modeling brain deformations in Alzheimer's disease by fluid registration of serial 3D MR images. J Comput Assist Tomogr 22:838–843

Freeborough PA, Woods RP, Fox NC (1996) Accurate registration of serial 3D MR brain images and its application to visualizing change in neurodegenerative disorders. J Comput Assist Tomogr 20:1012–1022

Friston KJ, Holmes AP, Worsley KJ, Poline J-P, Frith CD, Frackowiak RSJ (1995) Statistical parametric maps in functional imaging: a general linear approach. Human Brain Mapp 2:189–210

Hajnal JV, Saeed N, Soar EJ, Oatridge A, Young IR, Bydder GM (1995) A registration and interpolation procedure for subvoxel matching of serially acquired MR images. J Comput Assist Tomogr19:289–296

Jack CR Jr, Petersen RC, Xu YC, Waring SC, O'Brien PC, Tangalos EG, Smith GE, Ivnik RJ, Kokmen E (1997) Medial temporal atrophy on MRI in normal aging and very mild Alzheimer's disease. Neurology 49:786–794

Jack CR Jr, Petersen RC, Xu Y, O'Brien PC, Smith GE, Ivnik RJ, Tangalos EG, Kokmen E (1998) Rate of medial temporal lobe atrophy in typical aging and Alzheimer's disease. Neurology 51:993–999

Jack CR Jr, Petersen RC, Xu YC, O'Brien PC, Smith GE, Ivnik RJ, Boeve BF, Waring SC, Tangalos EG, Kokmen E (1999) Prediction of AD with MRI-based hippocampal volume in mild cognitive impairment. Neurology 52:1397–1403

Jack CR Jr, Slomkowski M, Gracon S, Hoover TM, Felmlee JP, Stewart K, Xu Y, Shiung M, O'Brien PC, Cha R, Knopman D, Petersen RC (2003) MRI as a biomarker of disease progression in a therapeutic trial of milameline for AD. Neurology 60:253–260

Janssen JC, Scahill RI, Schott JM, Whitwell JL, Stevens JM, Cipolotti L, Warrington EK, Rossor MN, Fox NC (2002) In vivo mapping of neurodegeneration in frontotemporal lobar degeneration. [Abstract]. Neurobiol Aging 23:S479

Leber P (1996) Observations and suggestions on antidementia drug development. Alzheimer Dis Assoc Disord 10:31–35

Lehericy S, Baulac M, Chiras J, Pierot L, Martin N, Pillon B, Deweer B,Dubois B, Marsault C (1994) Amygdalohippocampal MR volume measurements in the early stages of Alzheimer disease. Am J Neuroradiol 15:929–937

Rogers SL, Doody RS, Mohs RC, Friedhoff LT (1998) Donepezil improves cognition and global function in Alzheimer disease: a 15-week, double-blind, placebo-controlled study. Donepezil Study Group. Arch Int Med 158:1021–1031

Rosen WG, Mohs RC, Davis K (1984) A new rating scale for Alzheimer's disease. Am J Psychiat 141:1356–1364

Scahill RI, Schott JM, Stevens JM, Rossor MN, Fox NC (2002) Mapping the evolution of regional atrophy in Alzheimer's disease: unbiased analysis of fluid-registered serial MRI. Proc Natl Acad Sci (USA) 99:4703–4707

Scahill RI, Frost C, Jenkins R, Whitwell JL, Rossor MN, Fox NC (2003) A longitudinal study of brain volume changes in normal aging using serial registered magnetic resonance imaging. Arch Neurol, 60:989–994

Scheltens P, Fox NC, Barkhof F, DeCarli CD (2002) Structural magnetic resonance imaging in the practical assessment of dementia: beyond exclusion. Lancet Neurol 1:13–21

Schott JM, Fox NC, Frost C, Scahill RI, Janssen JC, Chan D, Jenkins R, Rossor MN (2003a) Assessing the onset of structural change in familial Alzheimer's disease. Ann Neurol 53:181–188

Schott JM, Simon JE, Fox NC, King AP, Khan MN, Cipolotti L, Paviour DC, Stevens JM, Rossor MN (2003b) Delineating the sites and progression of in vivo atrophy in multiple system atrophy using fluid-registered MRI Mov Disord 18:955–958

Schott JM, Simon JE, Whitwell JL, MacManus DG, Frost C, Wang L, Bartlett PA, Boyes RG, Rossor MN, Fox NC (2003c) Global brain atrophy as a surrogate marker of progression in Alzheimer's disease: a one year, prospective, longitudinal MRI study using the brain boundary shift integral. [Abstract]. Neurology 60 Supplement 1:A161

Woods RP, Grafton ST, Holmes CJ, Cherry SR, Mazziotta JC (1998) Automated image registration: I. General methods and intrasubject, intramodality validation. J Comput Assist Tomogr 22:139–152

Validating MRI Measures of Disease Stage and Progression in Alzheimer's Disease

Clifford R. Jack, Jr.[1]

Currently no absolute diagnostic marker exists for Alzheimer's disease (AD). Therefore, better non-invasive methods are needed to identify the risk of developing AD, staging the disease, and measuring its progression. The ideal biomarker would be a direct in vivo measurement of plaque and tangle burden, and promising results toward this objective have been reported in nuclear medicine (Klunk et al. 2002; Small et al. 2002). Until such direct measures have been thoroughly validated, however, other approaches must be employed. This chapter will review the literature supporting the position that indirect measures of AD can be valid biomarkers of disease stage and progression. It seems logical that indirect measures of disease can be valid biomarkers provided that changes in the measurement are empirically proven to track with independent measures of disease stage and progression, and that a plausible biological link exists between change in the measurement and progression of the disease itself. Magnetic resonance imaging (MRI) is a highly flexible imaging modality capable of measuring a number of different biologic parameters, for example, anatomic structure, metabolite concentration, proton diffusion, tissue perfusion, etc. All these tissue properties have been evaluated to some extent with MRI as potential diagnostic features of AD. The most widely studied MRI parameter in AD, however, is anatomic structure. Brain morphometry - specifically volume - is arguably the most straightforward of all tissue parameters measurable by MRI. Measurements of tissue volume are highly reliable and also have a strong, plausible biologic link to the pathologic progression of AD. In fact, loss of neurons and synaptic pruning, which are the substrates of cerebral atrophy, are felt to be more closely linked with the clinical progression of AD than plaque and tangle density (Fig. 1).

When measuring tissue volume with structural MRI, consideration must be given both to appropriate image acquisition and appropriate image analysis or post-processing methods. Image acquisition parameters must be selected to produce image volumes that appropriately capture the anatomic features of interest and are also technically suitable for the image processing methods proposed. For the most part, measurements of brain volume in AD are performed with high-resolution, three dimensional T1-weighted image volumes that can be acquired on any commercially available MRI scanner. Once appropriate images have been acquired, the image volumes may be processed in different ways to extract morphometric information. Methods of morphometric post processing can be divided into two major camps; segmentation and brain mapping. With the segmentation approach, the entire brain or individual brain structures are

---

[1] Department of Radiology, Mayo Clinic, 200 First Street SW Rochester, Minnesota U.S.A

Hyman et al.
The Living Brain and Alzheimer's
©Springer-Verlag Berlin Heidelberg

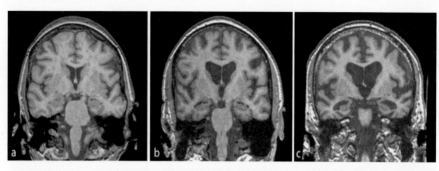

Fig. 1. Progressive atrophy with declining cognitive status.A-C, coronal T1-weighted images of a 70-year-old normal control, a 72-year-old MCI patient, and a 74-year-old AD patient, respectively. Notice the progressively more severe atrophy as cognitive status declines from normal to MCI to AD.

segmented from other brain regions and the number of voxels within the segmented region of interest is counted, leading to a direct measurement of tissue volume. The particular method of segmentation chosen depends largely on which anatomic structures are measured. For example, measurements of named medial temporal lobe structures – entorhinal cortex, hippocampus, etc. – have been the focus of much of the structural MRI work in AD due to the sequential nature of the pathologic progression of the disease. The initial neurofibrillary pathologic changes are found in the entorhinal cortex and hippocampus. Thus, MRI measurements designed to achieve early disease detection and measure pathologic progression early in the courses of the disease have focused on the medial temporal lobe. Because individual medial temporal lobe structures such as the hippocampus and entorhinal cortex do not have high contrast boundaries around their entire three-dimensional borders, the approach usually taken to measure the volume of these structures is manual tracing. Later progression of the disease is characterized by pathologic involvement that moves out of medial temporal limbic areas into association neocortex. MRI measurements of disease progression have, therefore, also focused on measures of whole brain atrophy. Measures of brain atrophy rates from serial MRI studies can be accomplished by individually segmenting the brain [or cerebrospinal fluid (CSF) spaces] on images acquired at baseline and at a later point(s) in time. Change in volume over time is measured by simple arithmetic subtraction of the individually derived volumes. Alternatively, image volumes can be spatially registered into a common anatomic coordinate system. The difference in volume between the images obtained at two different time points is then computed by one of several different methods: direct image subtraction, computation of intensity differences at the boundaries of the brain, or measurement of intensity gradients at the boundaries of the brain (Smith et al. 2002). The most widely studied approach in this category was developed by Fox and Freeborough (Fox and Freeborough 1997; Freeborough and Fox 1997) and is labeled the brain boundary shift integral method (BSI; Fig. 2). In addition to these methods, measurements of whole brain as well as of individual, targeted brain structures like the hippocampus have been performed using non-linear image

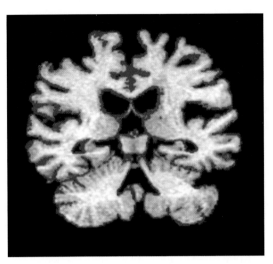

Fig. 2. Boundary shift integral in an AD patient. Volume loss at the brain-CSF interface between the two MRI studies, one year apart, is indicated by red pixels.

deformation algorithms with or without atlas-based templates (Freeborough and Fox 1998; Thompson et al. 1998, 2001, 2003; Studholme et al. 2001).

A second, fundamentally different approach to brain morphometry is voxel-based morphometry (Ashburner and Friston 2000; Davatzikos et al. 2001). In this approach, image volumes from different subjects are spatially normalized and morphometric parameters are calculated at each voxel position in the combined volume. For example, average gray matter concentration is calculated on a per voxel basis to derive estimates of regions of gray matter volume loss in one patient group relative to another (Baron et al. 2001; Chetelat et al. 2002; Karas et al. 2003). Regardless of the image-processing method employed, results have generally been quite consistent across studies published by a number of different groups. Structural MRI measures do seem to be valid biomarkers of disease stage and progression. In the remainder of this chapter, the literature supporting structural MRI as a valid biomarker will be reviewed. The pertinent literature can be considered under several different categories, depending on the type of clinical study employed: cross-sectional MRI-clinical correlation; MRI-autopsy correlation; predicting future development of AD; and measures of atrophy rates from serial MRI.

Cross-sectional MRI-Clinical Correlation

The first step in validating the clinical utility of an imaging method is to document correlations between imaging and clinical status in cross-sectional case-control studies. In AD, this initial step involves testing the hypothesis that an imaging measurement is significantly different between patients with clinically established AD and appropriately matched controls. The argument is sometimes made that this type of cross-sectional, case control study fails to document any added diagnostic value for imaging – because the gold standard against which imaging is compared is the clinical diagnosis of normality or AD, both of which are available through the clinical examination. In fact, however, this type of cross-sectional, case control study is an essential step in validating the clinical utility of any new imaging test, because if the imaging study failed to pass this most basic test of diagnostic utility, there would be little sense in pursing more demanding clinical applications. Cross-sectional, case control data are arguably the most readily accessible type of imaging correlation data to obtain. As a result, the vast majority of the literature published on AD to date has been of the cross-sectional, case control variety. Because of the large number of studies published at this point, individual studies will not be reviewed here. In general, however, structural MRI measures seem to match the clinical stage of the disease, with atrophy of the entorhinal cortex and hippocampus evident earliest and most severely, and with involvement of the neocortex later in disease progression. There is nearly universal agreement that structural MRI measures are different between patients with established AD and appropriately matched control subjects. This is true in the earliest stages of AD as well, with several studies documenting significant differences between normal subjects and patients with mild cognitive impairment. While respectable diagnostic sensitivity and specificity have been reported from numerous groups in separating controls from patients with mild AD or patients with MCI, nearly every study has also found overlap between the patient and control groups. Precise sensitivity and specificity for diagnostic intergroup separation vary among different studies. Often differences in sensitivity and specificity are attributed to technical aspects of measurement. For example, studies have appeared in the literature arguing that measures of the hippocampus are more sensitive than measurements of the temporal lobe, that measurements of the entorhinal cortex are more sensitive than measures of the hippocampus, that one method of entorhinal or hippocampal measurement is superior to another, etc.

While the technical aspects of the measurement technique certainly play a role in diagnostic sensitivity and specificity, an underappreciated reason for differences in results among groups is that the research subjects themselves are different. Among the various published studies, different criteria have been used to define normality, different criteria have been used to define mild cognitive impairment, the ages of study groups have varied sometimes dramatically, study subjects have been drawn from community samples in some and from referral samples in other studies, etc. The emphasis in the literature tends to focus on the inherent diagnostic sensitivity and specificity of a particular measurement technique. But, in reality, in order to perform a truly valid comparison of diagnostic sensitivity and specificity of different measurement methods, the techniques must be compared in the same subjects.

Autopsy-MRI Correlations

The most convincing evidence validating an imaging measurement technique as a legitimate biomarker of disease stage is the imaging-pathology correlation. This type of data is not readily available and, as a result, few such studies have appeared in the literature. However, the data that have appeared in the literature do seem to validate that quantitative MRI measurements are a reasonable reflection of pathologic disease stage in AD. Bobinski et al. (2000) performed post-mortem MRI studies of fixed brain specimens. Hippocampal volumes were measured from the resulting post-mortem MRI images. These MRI measures were correlated with histologic measurements of hippocampal area and neuronal cell counts, and highly significant MRI-histology correlations were found. Our group performed a study correlating measures of hippocampal volume from ante-mortem MRI studies with post-mortem assessments of disease stage (Jack et al. 2002). Pathologic staging was performed using the method of Braak and Braak (Braak et al. 1993) in an unselected series of 67 individuals. A many AD subjects, we found significant correlations (all p<0.01) between ante-mortem hippocampal volume and Braak stage (R = –.63), between hippocampal volume and last ante-mortem MMSE score (R = –.41), and between MMSE score and Braak stage (R = –.61). In this same study, significant hippocampal atrophy was seen in subjects who were demented due to non-AD conditions such as frontotemporal dementia, hippocampal sclerosis, etc. Therefore, brain atrophy is certainly not specific for AD. However, both our results and those of Bobinski et al. (2000) indicate that, in patients who lie along the pathologic continuum from normality to AD, the degree of atrophy, in this case of the hippocampus, is an approximate indicator of pathologic stage.

Predicting Development of AD

In each person who develops AD, the transition from normal to clearly recognizable AD occurs gradually over a number of years, without an abrupt transition point. It is widely presumed that the pathologic substrate of the cognitive decline that characterizes AD follows a similar course, with progressive accumulation of degenerative pathology ongoing for years prior to manifestation of any obvious clinical symptoms. Given the slow nature of pathologic progression, therefore, the concept of early diagnosis can be recast in AD as predicting the risk of developing the clinical syndrome. The optimal subjects in whom to intervene therapeutically are those who are destined to develop AD but who do not yet manifest any clinical symptoms – actually, in subjects who have no pathologic changes of AD at all. With the anticipated arrival of disease-modifying therapeutic interventions, there is great interest in identifying markers that accurately predict the future development of AD. Operationally, predicting future development of AD can be thought of in two stages: predicting conversion from normality to mild cognitive impairment, and predicting conversion of MCI to AD. An antecedent biomarker is one that predicts future development of MCI in subjects who are currently asymptotic. Identifying and clinically validating such an antecedent biomarker would be quite difficult logistically. In theory, a study validating an antecedent biomarker would need to enroll a cohort of individuals in their 30s or 40s, measure the biomarker of interest, and then follow the cohort for decades in order to prove the hypothesis that the biomarker did indeed predict the future development of AD. An alternative approach has been employed in nuclear medicine, where glucose metabolism patterns of asymptomatic APOE4 carriers have been contrasted with those of APOE4 non-carriers (Reiman et al. 1996; Small et al. 2000). Evidence resulting from these studies is certainly suggestive, as APOE4 carriers are much more likely to develop AD in the future than are E4 non-carriers. However, this type of cross-sectional study design cannot be considered to truly validate an antecedent biomarker.

Validating a biomarker of secondary progression, that is progression from MCI to AD, is a much more tractable problem, and these types of studies have been performed with MRI. The study design involves acquiring a baseline MRI study from which volume measurements of some structure or structures are measured in a cohort of individuals with MCI. The cohort of MCI subjects is then followed longitudinally to test the hypothesis that the baseline MRI measurement predicts subsequent conversion to AD over a defined period of time. More precisely, the hypothesis being tested is that a baseline MRI measurement can predict the rate at which individuals with MCI will convert to AD. Several groups have published on this topic. Baseline volumetric measurements of several different anatomic structures have been shown to predict conversion from mild impairment to AD, including the hippocampus (Kaye et al. 1997; Jack et al. 1999), entorhinal cortex (Dickerson et al. 2001; Killiany et al. 2002), medial temporal lobe (Visser et al. 1999), temporal lobe (Kaye et al. 1997), middle temporal and inferior temporal gyri, and the caudal portion of the anterior cingulate gyrus (Killiany et al. 2000; Fig. 3). Visual assessment of medial temporal lobe atrophy has also shown predictive power (de Leon et al. 1993). In addition, accelerated rates of whole brain and hippocampal atrophy have been identified in presymptomatic individuals with an autosomal dominant APP mutation that were destined to later develop AD (Fox et al. 1999, 2001; Schott et al. 2003).

Atrophy Rate Measures from Serial MRI

Clinical/behavioral measures are employed to assess disease progression in individual patients for clinical purposes and also are the standard method for assessing therapeutic efficacy in AD drug trials. However, the high test-re-test variability of clinical/behavioral measures has led many in academia and industry to consider rates of change in imaging measures as biomarkers of disease progression. Some data are available indicating that serial measures of glucose metabolism from FDG PET may be useful (Small et al. 2000; Reiman et al. 2001). In MRI, the two imaging measures that have received the most attention are measures of the rates of change in whole brain volume and hippocampal volume. Longitudinal imaging data are arguably some of the most difficult data to come by, for several reasons. First, technical demands are high. The technical stability of the MRI scan or scanners used to image study subjects serially must be maintained at a constant level over a number of years. For example, the key indices in MRI are measures of the geometric fidelity of the individual MRI scanners and contrast to noise. These parameters must be measured at regular intervals and, when a scanner begins to deviate from pre-specified specifications, it must be re-calibrated. This procedure is particularly true for geometric fidelity, which tends to drift in MRI, particularly with hardware or software upgrades. Second, the type of clinical

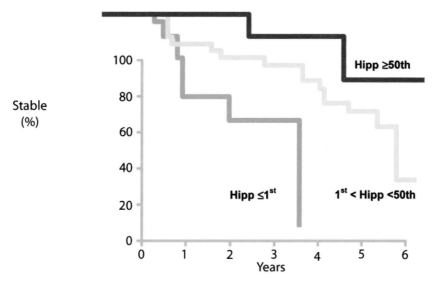

Fig. 3. Hippocampal volume at baseline and subsequent conversion from MCI to AD. MCI subjects without atrophy at baseline – with hippocampal volumes ≥50th percentile of normal – were less likely to convert to AD than MCIs with more atrophic hippocompi.

study necessary to validate atrophy rate measures from serial MRI as legitimate biomarkers of disease progression is logistically complex. Patients must be enrolled and scanned at baseline. Subjects then must be followed by clinical and MRI assessments at predetermined intervals over a span of at least several years. A minimum of three to five years is required to enroll and serially study a group of subjects large enough to extract meaningful data. For this reason, relatively few studies have appeared in the literature to date on the topic of measuring rates of atrophy from serial MRI. However, this is beginning to change, and the data that have been published uniformly demonstrate that atrophy rates do differ between patients and controls and that the test-re-test precision of imaging measures seems to be superior to standard clinical and behavioral measures.

Several different types of studies have been published in this area. Rates of whole brain and hippocampal atrophy in AD patients with an autosomal dominant APP mutation exceed those in appropriately matched controls. This finding has been documented with different measurement techniques, including boundary shift integral measures of whole brain, hippocampal tracing, and a method to forward propagate hippocampal segmentation with non-linear deformation type registration (Fox et al. 1996, 2001; Crum et al. 2001). Among the very old, rates of hippocampal atrophy in AD patients are greater than those in age-matched control subjects (Kaye et al. 1997; Jack et al. 1998). In typical late-onset AD, rates of atrophy of the hippocampus and entorhinal cortex in AD subjects exceed those in age-matched controls (Jack et al. 1998; Du et al. 2003). Rates of sulcal and ventricular enlargement in typical late-onset AD exceed those in normal controls (Jack et al. 1998; Thompson et al. 2001).

A second type of serial MRI study asks the question, "Do rates of atrophy on imaging match clinical change over time?" Given a group of normal controls and a group of MCI patients enrolled at baseline, some of the normal controls and some of the MCI subjects will decline cognitively over the period of observation. Normal controls may convert to MCI, and MCI subjects may convert to AD over the interval of time that the serial MRI studies are acquired. Using clinical group transition (over lack thereof) as the independent, gold standard measure of disease progression, one can test the hypothesis that rates of change on imaging correlate with clinical progression over time. Such a study has been performed with serial MR measures of the hippocampus (Jack et al. 2000; Table 1). In this study, annualized rates of hippocampal atrophy were 1.7% per year for controls who remained stable vs 2.8% per year for controls who declined to MCI and 2.5% per year for MCIs who remained stable vs 3.7% per year for MCIs who declined to AD. The observed rates of hippocampal atrophy match clinical change or lack of clinical change within each of the baseline groups very well. From this study one can conclude that rates of hippocampal atrophy do match change in cognitive status (or lack thereof) over time in elderly persons who lie along the cognitive continuum from normal to MCI to AD.

Most of the MRI work published to date has consisted of single-site studies. Technical challenges in terms of insuring MRI data quality, data storage, data handling, etc., while demanding at single sites, are considerably greater when dealing with multi-site data. A logical question, therefore, is, can the positive results that have been reported from several different groups at single sites be demonstrated using multi-site data. A recent study demonstrates the technical feasibility of multi-site MRI studies in AD (Jack et al. 2003). This study began as a therapeutic trial of Milameline, a cholinergic agonist. The study was designed as a 52-week controlled trial with an enrollment of 450 AD subjects, all in the mild to moderate phase of the disease. The therapeutic trial itself was not completed due to projected lack of efficacy on interim analysis. However, the MRI arm of the study was continued in a subset of subjects, thus effectively converting what began as a therapeutic trial into a natural history observational study of AD. A total of 192 subjects from 38 different centers ultimately underwent two MRI studies at a one-year interval. From these data, rates of change of hippocampal and temporal horn volume were measured. Change from baseline behavioral cognitive and MRI variables in these 192 subjects are indicated in Table 2. The annual raw and annual percentage changes in ADAS-Cog and MMSE are fairly typical for AD patients with mild to moderate disease. Annual change in hippocampal and temporal horn volume were in close agreement with values published earlier from a

Table 1. Percent annual change in hippocampal volume by follow-up clinical group[a]

Control-Stable (N=48)	-1,7 ± 0,9
Control-Decliner (N=10)	-2,8 ± 1,7
MCI-Stable (N=25)	-2,5 ± 1,5
MCI-Decliner (N=18)	-3,7 ± 1,5
AD (N=28)	-3,5 ± 1,8

[a] Values in table represent mean ± SD (range).

Table 2. Change from baseline in behavioral/cognitive and MRI variables

	Annual raw change (N=192)	Annual % change (N=192)	Percent decliners
ADAS-Cog	4,1	16,4	60
MMSE	– 1,9	– 8,4	64
GDS	0	0,0	38
Total hippocampal mm^3	– 221	– 4,9	99
Total temporal horn volume mm^3	616	16,1	85

single site (Jack et al. 1998, 2000). Of interest, however, was the percentage of AD patients who declined over time on these various measures. Less than two-thirds of these AD subjects declined over a one-year period of time on the ADAS-Cog and MMSE, and only about one-third declined on the GDS. In contrast, hippocampal volume declined in 99% of subjects and the temporal horns enlarged in 85%. Power calculations were performed on these data. Assuming a 50% effect size (i.e., rate reduction over one year), the number of subjects per arm needed to power the study using the ADAS-Cog was 320, for the MMSE 241, for the temporal horn volume 54, and hippocampal volume 21. The substantially smaller sample sizes required for imaging vs. standard clinical/behavioral measures were due to the fact that the imaging measures declined more consistently across the study group than did the behavioral/cognitive measures. Fox et al. (2000) also demonstrated that a significant reduction in sample size is possible using measures of whole brain atrophy with the boundary shift integral method when compared to standard clinical/behavioral measures.

The best available evidence supporting the validity of MRI as a biomarker of disease progression is multiple, independent, natural history studies that consistently demonstrate concordant MRI and clinical change over time. The studies cited above meet this criterion. A distinction should be borne in mind between validating MRI as a biomarker of disease progression vs. validating serial MRI as a surrogate measure of therapeutic efficacy. The former can be accomplished with the types of natural history studies cited above. Validating MRI as an appropriate surrogate outcome measure for trials of therapeutic efficacy must await a positive, disease-modifying therapeutic trial that has incorporated MRI.

References

Ashburner J, Friston KJ (2000) Voxel-based morphometry--the methods. NeuroImage 11: 805–821

Baron JC, Chetelat G, Desgranges B, Perchey G, Landeau B, de la Sayette V, Eustache F (2001) In vivo mapping of gray matter loss with voxel-based morphometry in mild Alzheimer's disease. Neuroimage 14: 298–309

Bobinski M, de Leon MJ, Wegiel J, Desanti S, Convit A, Saint Louis LA, Rusinek H, Wisniewski HM (2000) The histological validation of post mortem magnetic resonance imaging-determined hippocampal volume in Alzheimer's disease. Neuroscience 95: 721–725

Braak H, Braak E, Bohl J (1993) Staging of Alzheimer-related cortical destruction. Eur Neurol 33: 403–408.

Chetelat G, Desgranges B, De La Sayette V, Viader F, Eustache F, Baron JC (2002) Mapping gray matter loss with voxel-based morphometry in mild cognitve impairment. Brain Imaging 13: 1939

Crum, WR, Scahill RI, Fox NC (2001) Automated hippocampal segmentation by regional fluid registration of serial MRI: validation and application in Alzheimer's disease. Neuroimage 13: 847–855

de Leon MJ, Golomb J, George AE, Convit A, Tarshish CY, McRae T, De Santi S, Smith G, Ferris SH, Noz M (1993) The radiologic prediction of Alzheimer disease: the atrophic hippocampal formation. AJNR 14: 897–906

Dickerson BC, Goncharova I, Sullivan MP, Forchetti C, Wilson RS, Bennett DA, Beckett LA, de-Toledo-Morrell L (2001) MRI-derived entorhinal and hippocampal atrophy in incipient and very mild Alzheimer's disease. Neurobiol Aging 22: 747–754

Du AT, Schuff N, Zhu XP, Jagust WJ, Miller BL, Reed BR, Kramer JH, Mungas D, Yaffe K, Chui HC, Weiner MW (2003) Atrophy rates of entorhinal cortex in AD and normal aging. Neurology 60: 481–486.

Fox NC, Freeborough PA (1997) Brain atrophy progression measured from registered serial MRI: validation and application to Alzheimer's disease. J Magnetic Resonance Imaging 7: 1069–1075

Fox NC, Warrington EK, Freeborough PA, Hartikainen P, Kennedy AM, Stevens JM, Rossor MN (1996) Presymptomatic hippocampal atrophy in Alzheimer's disease. A longitudinal MRI study. Brain 119: 2001–2007

Fox NC, Warrington EK, Rossor MN (1999) Serial magnetic resonance imaging of cerebral atrophy in preclinical Alzheimer's disease. Lancet 353: 2125

Fox NC, Cousens S, Scahill R, Harvey RJ, Rossor MN (2000) Using serial registered brain magnetic resonance imaging to measure disease progression in Alzheimer disease. Arch Neurol 57: 339–443

Fox NC, Crum WR, Scahill RI, Stevens JM, Janssen JC, Rossor MN (2001) Imaging of onset and progression of Alzheimer's disease with voxel-compression mapping of serial magnetic resonance images. Lancet 358: 201–205

Freeborough PA, Fox NC (1997) The boundary shift integral: an accurate and robust measure of cerebral volume changes from registered repeat MRI. IEEE Trans Med Imaging 15: 623–629

Freeborough PA, Fox NC (1998) Modeling brain deformations in Alzheimer's disease by fluid registration of serial 3D MRI. JCAT 22: 838–843

Jack CR Jr, Petersen RC, Xu Y, O'Brien PC, Smith GE, Ivnik RJ, Tangalos EG, Kokmen E (1998) The rate of medial temporal lobe atrophy in typical aging and Alzheimer's disease. Neurology 51: 993–999

Jack CR Jr, Petersen RC, Xu YC, O'Brien PC, Smith GE, Ivnik RJ, Boeve BF, Waring SC, Tangalos EG, Kokmen E (1999) Prediction of AD with MRI-based hippocampal volume in mild cognitive impairment. Neurology 52: 1397–1403

Jack CR Jr, Petersen RC, Xu Y, O'Brien PC, Smith GE, Ivnik RJ, Boeve BF, Tangalos EG, Kokmen E (2000) Rates of hippocampal atrophy in normal aging, mild cognitive impairment, and Alzheimer's disease. Neurology 55: 484–489

Jack CR Jr, Dickson DW, Parisi JE, Xu YC, Cha RH, O'Brien PC, Edland SD, Smith GE, Boeve BF, Tangalos EG, Kokmen E, Petersen RC (2002) Antemortem MRI findings correlate with hippocampal neuropathology in typical aging and dementia. Neurology 58: 750–757

Jack CR Jr, Slomkowski M, Gracon S, Hoover TM, Felmlee JP, Stewart K, Xu Y, Shiung M, O'Brien PC, Cha R, Knopman D, Petersen RC (2003) MRI as a biomarker of disease progression in a therapeutic trial of Milameline for Alzheimer's. Neurology 60: 253–260

Karas GB, Burton EJ, Rombouts SA, van Schijndel RA, O'Brien JT, Scheltens P, McKeith IG, Williams D, Ballard C, Barkhof F (2003) A comprehensive study of gray matter loss in patients with Alzheimer's disease using optimized voxel-based morphometry. NeuroImage 18: 895–907

Kaye JA, Swihart T, Howieson D, Dame A, Moore MM, Karnos T, Camicioli R, Ball M, Oken B, Sexton G (1997) Volume loss of the hippocampus and temporal lobe in healthy elderly persons destined to develop dementia. Neurology 48: 1297–1304

Killiany RJ, Gomez-Isla T, Moss M, Kikinis R, Sandor T, Jolesz F, Tanzi R, Jones K, Hyman BT, Albert MS (2000) Use of structural magnetic resonance imaging to predict who will get Alzheimer's disease. Ann Neurol 47: 430–439

Killiany RJ, Hyman BT, Gomez-Isla T, Moss MB, Kikinis R, Jolesz F, Tanzi R, Jones K, Albert MS (2002) MRI measures of entorhinal cortex vs hippomcampus in preclinical AD. Neurology 58: 1188–1196

Klunk WE, Bacskai BJ, Mathis CA, Kajdasz ST, McLellan ME, Frosch MP, Debnath ML, Holt DP, Wang Y, Hyman BT (2002) Imaging A-beta plaques in living transgenic mice with multiphoton microscopy and methoxy-X04, a systemically administered congo red derivative. J Neuropathol Exp Neurol 61: 797–805

Reiman EM, Caselli RJ, Chen K, Alexander GE, Bandy D, Frost J (2001) Declining brain activity in cognitively normal apolipoprotein E E4 heterozygotes: a foundation for using positron emission tomography to efficiently test treatments to prevent Alzheimer's disease. Proc Natl Acad Sci USA 98: 3334–3339

Reiman EM, Caselli RJ, Yun LS, Chen K, Bandy D, Minoshima S, Thibodeau SN, Osborne D (1996) Preclinical evidence of Alzheimer's disease in persons homozygous for the E4 allele for apolipoprotein E. New Engl J Med334: 752–758

Schott JM, Fox NC, Frost C, Scahill RI, Janssen JC, Chan D, Jenkins R, Rossor MN (2003) Assessing the onset of structural change in familial Alzheimer's disease. Ann Neurol 53: 181–188

Small GW, Ercoli LM, Silverman DH, Huang SC, Komo S, Bookheimer SY, Lavretsky H, Miller K, Siddarth P, Rasgon NL, Mazziotta JC, Saxena S, Wu HM, Mega MS, Cummings JL, Saunders AM, Pericak-Vance MA, Roses AD, Barrio JR, Phelps ME (2000). Cerebral metabolic and cognitive decline in persons at genetic risk for Alzheimer's disease. Proc Natl Acad Sci USA 87: 6037–6042

Small GW, Agdeppa ED, Kepe V, Satyamurthy N, Huang SC, Barrio JR (2002) In vivo brain imaging of tangle burden in humans. J Mol Neurosci19: 323–327

Studholme C, Cardenas V, Schuff N, Rosen H, Miller B, Weiner M (2001) Detecting spatially consistent structural differences in Alzheimer's and fronto temporal dementia using deformation morphometry. p 41–44.MICCAI 4th International Conference, Utrecht, The Netherlands, Springer

Thompson PM, Moussai J, Zohoori S, Goldkorn A, Khan AA, Mega MS, Small GW, Cummings JL, Toga AW (1998) Cortical variability and asymmetry in normal aging and Alzheimer's disease. Cereb Cortex 8: 492–509

Thompson PM, Mega MS, Woods RP, Zoumalan CI, Lindshield CJ, Blanton RE, Moussai J, Holmes CJ, Cummings JL, Toga AW (2001) Cortical change in Alzheimer's disease detected with a disease-specific population-based brain atlas. Cereb Cortex 11: 1–16

Thompson P, Rapoport JL, Cannon TD, Toga AW (2003) Automated analysis of structural MRI data. In: Lawrie EJS, Weinberger D (eds) Brain imaging in schizophrenia. Oxford, Oxford University Press, pp 1–36

Visser PJ, Scheltens P, Verhey FR, Schmand B, Launer LJ, Jolles J, Jonker C (1999) Medial temporal lobe atrophy and memory dysfunction as predictors for dementia in subjects with mild cognitive impairment. J Neurol 246: 477–485

Dynamic Mapping of Alzheimer's Disease

Paul M. Thompson[1], Kiralee M. Hayashi[1], Greig de Zubicaray[2], Andrew L. Janke[2], Elizabeth R. Sowell[1], Stephen E. Rose[2], James Semple[3], David Herman[1], Michael S. Hong[1], Stephanie S. Dittmer[1], David M. Doddrell[2], Arthur W. Toga[1]

Summary

Neuroimaging strategies to track Alzheimer's disease are greatly accelerating our understanding of the disease. How early can we detect disease-related brain changes? How do these changes progress anatomically? Do drugs slow down the physical spread of the disease? Brain imaging now provides answers to some of these important questions. With recent innovations in magnetic resonance imaging (MRI) and brain image analysis, Alzheimer's disease can be mapped dynamically as it spreads in the living brain (Reiman et al. 2001; Fox et al. 2001; Janke et al. 2001; Thompson et al. 2003a). Drug and gene effects on the disease process can be detected, both in patients and in family members at increased genetic risk. We show how these brain mapping tools help explore the dynamic processes of aging and dementia, revealing factors that affect them. As an illustrative example, we report the mapping of a dynamically spreading wave of gray matter loss in the brains of Alzheimer's patients scanned repeatedly with MRI. The loss pattern is visualized, in 3D, as it spreads from temporal cortices into frontal and cingulate brain regions. Deficit patterns are resolved with a novel cortical pattern matching strategy (CPM). A dynamic mapping technique produces color-coded image sequences that reveal the disease spreading in the human cortex over a period of several years. The trajectory of cortical deficits, observed here in vivo with MRI, corresponded closely to the spread of the underlying pathology (as defined by the well-known Braak stages of neurofibrillary tangle and beta-amyloid accumulation). The magnitude of these deficits was also tightly linked with cognitive decline. In initial studies, these maps detected disease effects more sensitively than conventional cortical anatomic volume measures. By storing these dynamic brain maps in a growing, population-based digital atlas ($N>1000$ subjects), clinical imaging data can be analyzed on a large scale, adjusting for effects of age, sex, genotype, and disease subtypes. These maps chart the dynamic progress of Alzheimer's disease and reveal a changing pattern of cortical deficits. We are now

[1] Laboratory of Neuro Imaging, Brain Mapping Division, Department of Neurology, UCLA School of Medicine, 710 Westwood Plaza, Los Angeles, CA 90095, USA
[2] Centre for Magnetic Resonance, University of Queensland, Brisbane, Australia
[3] GlaxoSmithKline Pharmaceuticals plc, Addenbrooke's Centre for Clinical Investigation, Addenbrooke's Hospital, Hills Road, CB2 2GG, Cambridge, UK

using them to detect where deficit patterns are modified by drug treatment and known risk genotypes.

Introduction

Impact of Alzheimer's Disease

Alzheimer's disease (AD) is a severe and growing public health crisis. The disease causes irreversible memory loss, behavioral and cognitive decline, personality changes, and a decreasing ability to cope with everyday life. The incidence of AD within the population doubles every five years after age 60, afflicting 1% of those aged 60 to 64 and 30–40% of those aged 85 and older. Without a cure, the number of AD victims will rise from 2 to 3.5 million now to an estimated 10–14 million by the year 2030 (Malmgren 2000). A number of promising AD treatments are now being developed. These range from acetylcholinesterase inhibitors, which ballast neurotransmitter function, to vaccines, which directly attack the amyloid plaques that are a key element of AD pathology (Forette et al. 2002). Most therapeutic trials of new drugs in AD rely on brief cognitive testing to determine efficacy (Grundman et al. 2002; Jack et al. 2003). Because the brief and sometimes non-standardized cognitive measures used in clinical trials are notoriously variable, neuroimaging can be extremely beneficial in this research. Brain imaging may eventually help us quantify how AD emerges, even before cognitive symptoms appear, and chart how the disease spreads in the brain. With the continuing development of new treatments, neuroimaging supplies a variety of biological markers that measure disease progress. These measures can be collected from large numbers of patients in clinical trials. Dynamic brain mapping strategies, described in this paper, are particularly well-suited to evaluate new therapies, because they allow us to track the disease process in exquisite detail, as it spreads in the living brain.

Goals of Neuroimaging

Depending on the goals of the study, a wide variety of neuroimaging measures can be used to characterize dementia (Black 1999; Chetelat and Baron 2003). For instance, MRI data can provide sensitive quantitative measures of the cerebral cortex and can assess the integrity of medial temporal lobe structures involved in memory. The required 3D MRI scans can be performed in approximately 10 minutes, on a conventional 1.5 Tesla scanner. Ultimately, our goal is to use the brain imaging data to 1) screen at-risk populations, to estimate each individual's likelihood of developing AD; 2) discriminate AD from normal aging and other dementias (such as frontotemporal and Lewy body dementias); and 3) monitor disease progress and therapeutic response. Early detection of the disease is vital because cholinergic drugs are most effective in the mildest phases, when widespread neuronal loss has not yet occurred. Up to 30 years elapse between the onset of AD pathology (neurofibrillary tangles and neuritic plaques) and clinical changes that suggest a diagnosis (Braak and Braak 1997; Ohm et al. 1995; Thal et al. 2002). Imaging technology has emerged that is safe, repeatable, and widely available and can track dynamic brain changes over the human life span. These changes can be evaluated prospectively, with a variety of biomarkers derived from brain images (Haller et al. 1997; Csernansky et al. 2000; Resnick et al. 2000; Bartzokis et al. 2001; Crum et al. 2001; O'Brien et al. 2001; Chan et al. 2001; Davatizkos et al. 2001, 2002; Studholme et al. 2001; Ge et al. 2002; Miller et al. 2002; Scheltens et al. 2002; Smith 2002; Rosen et al. 2002; Wang et al. 2002; Thompson et al. 2003a; Ashburner et al. 2003). The region and rate of atrophic brain changes in dementia can be measured with such methods. While MRI is not currently used in the diagnosis of AD, the new technology in brain image analysis provides great promise for better discriminating AD from normal aging and for tracking how medications affect the path of the disease in the brain.

Repeated Scanning Over Time

In the 1990s, MRI research in dementia focused on measuring medial temporal lobe structures (Jobst et al. 1992, 1994; Jack et al. 1992, 1997, 1998; De Leon et al. 1997; Fox et al. 1996). This was because Alzheimer pathology typically starts in the temporal cortex adjacent to the entorhinal cortex and quickly spreads to the entorhinal cortex before involving the hippocampus (Braak and Braak 1997; Frisoni et al. 1999; Laakso et al. 2000a, b; Dickerson et al. 2001). This temporal lobe pathology persists for several years (Smith 2002) before spreading cortically to engulf the rest of the temporal, frontal, and parietal lobes (Braak and Braak 1997; Thal et al. 2002; Thompson et al. 2001b, 2003b). A more recent trend in dementia research has been to move from cross-sectional studies to dynamic measures. This approach can increase the power to resolve group and treatment effects (Jack et al. 2003). Serial MRI scans (i.e., acquired from the same patients repeatedly over time) can provide much greater power to detect pathological atrophy, as they provide a baseline reference point to calculate change. A key limitation with single time-point measures is their poor power to detect incipient disease processes. The large inter- and intra-individual variability in brain structure leads to an overlap of AD and normal aging, for most simple volumetric measures made at any single time point. Demonstration of *deteriorating* brain structure, especially when linked with cognitive or metabolic decline, has greater prognostic value. Such changes almost certainly reflect progression of underlying brain pathology.

Brain Tissue Loss

In early work, Fox and colleagues (1996) found that AD patients lose brain tissue *overall*, at a faster rate than age-matched controls, in MRI scans acquired one year apart (Fox et al. 1996, 1997, 2000; Rossor et al. 1997; Scahill et al. 2002). Evaluated with MRI for five to eight years, AD patients lost brain tissue at a median rate of 2.20% per year (range 0.82 to 4.19) versus 0.24% per year in controls (range -0.35 to 0.64; $p<0.0001$; Fox et al. 2001). These rates correlated with the rate of decline in MMSE scores (Mini Mental State Exam; Folstein 1975). Using volume measures, Bradley et al. (2002) studied 39 elderly subjects with serial MRI over three- to six-month intervals. They measured the ratio of the ventricular volume to the total brain volume (i.e., the ventricle-to-brain ratio; VBR). The VBR rate of change was 15.6% ± 2.8% (mean ± SD) per year for probable AD compared with 4.3% ± 1.1% per year for negative AD ($p<0.0001$). VBR did not separate groups when measured at only a single time point, supporting the value of longitudinal assessments. Power calculations revealed that 135 subjects would be needed in each arm of a placebo-controlled clinical trial if this measure of disease progression were to detect a 20% reduction in the excess rate of atrophy over 6 months, with 90% power.

From Volumes to Maps

While *volumes* of brain structures provide simple, useful measures of atrophy, *maps* of atrophic processes provide additional advantages. Brain maps can uncover the spatial profile of anatomical change in serially imaged populations. They can help us visualize the spatial patterns of tissue deficits, rates of cortical atrophy, and subtle anatomical shape changes throughout the entire brain. Maps of atrophy can isolate regions where brain change is fastest and can reveal how the disease spreads through the cortex over a period of several years (Janke et al. 2001; Thompson et al. 2001b,c; 2003b). When statistics of these changes are stored in a digital brain atlas, statistical criteria can be used to identify regions where atrophic rates differ across clinical groups (Thompson et al. 2001b, c), such as those receiving different medications.

Overview of this Paper

This paper describes these mapping approaches. We focus on understanding how the cortex changes in AD. Specialized algorithms map the progressive impact of AD as it spreads, allowing us to visualize brain changes in animation (Thompson et al. 2003a). We use examples to show how brain mapping techniques have revealed new information on the processes of aging and dementia. They have mapped how the cortex changes across the human life span (Sowell et al. 2003; n=176 subjects), how it differs in disorders such as schizophrenia (Thompson et al. 2001f) and fetal alcohol syndrome (Sowell et al. 2002), and how genetic differences influence these changes (Thompson et al. 2001a, 2002c). The resulting maps and statistics can provide powerful criteria to differentiate normal from abnormal brain change and can be used to identify factors that affect the course of aging and dementia. We also describe some specialized image analysis algorithms that maximize the statistical power of these analyses and make it easier to localize deficit patterns in a group. The resulting brain mapping tools provide quantitative predictors to monitor brain degeneration and gauge how well it is decelerated or delayed in clinical trials.

Computational Anatomy: Applications to AD

Extreme intersubject variations in brain structure hinder our ability to understand what brain changes generally occur as a patient develops Alzheimer's disease. Without methods to overcome the problems of anatomic variability, the statistical power to resolve disease and treatment effects is seriously undermined. First, normal anatomical variation results in an overlapping of diseased and normal subjects on most anatomical measures. Second, although AD is primarily a cortical disease, wide variations in gyral and sulcal features make it difficult to combine data across subjects whose anatomy is different. These difficulties are exacerbated in AD by disease-related atrophy (Meltzer and Frost 1994; Woods 1996; Mega et al. 1997; Thompson et al. 1998). Finally, profiles of gray matter loss are difficult to calibrate against a reference population, due to the lack of statistics on expected changes in elderly populations. To fully capitalize on neuroimaging data in AD, an appropriately complex mathematical framework is needed to address these three challenges. Once resolved, brain maps can then be compared across patients and across time (Mazziotta et al. 1995; Thompson et al. 1997a, b; 2000a, b; Grenander and Miller 1998)

Maps of Gray Matter Deficits in Alzheimer's Disease

In our early MRI studies, we set out to determine the pattern of gray matter loss in mild to moderate AD, relative to matched healthy controls (Thompson et al. 2001b). In early AD, intraneuronal filamentous deposits, or neurofibrillary tangles (NFTs), accumulate within neurons. These deposits are composed of hyperphosphorylated tau-protein (Hulstaert et al. 1999). This cellular pathology disrupts axonal transport and induces widespread metabolic decline; it eventually leads to neuronal loss, observed as gross atrophy on MRI. Braak and Braak (1997) noted at autopsy that NFT distribution was initially restricted to entorhinal cortices, spreading to higher order temporo-parietal association cortices, then to frontal, and ultimately primary sensory and visual areas (cf. Delacourte et al. 1999; Price and Morris 1999). We set out to determine whether a similar wave of cortical atrophy could be mapped in patients while they were alive. The goal was to visualize the disease's transit within cortex and relate it to cognitive decline.

Analysis Pipeline

Figure 1 shows a sequence of image processing steps used to do this (Thompson et al. 2003a). This image analysis pipeline can be applied, in general, to MRI brain scans to understand how the cortex is affected in disease. The analysis can also reveal where anatomic differences (e.g., local gray matter losses) are linked with measures of cognitive decline, genotype, or medication effects, as well as demographic variables such as age and gender. The mathematics of these techniques are covered elsewhere (Thompson and Toga 2002) but are briefly described here.

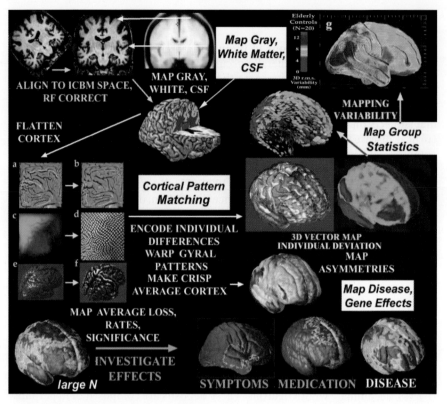

Fig. 1. Analyzing cortical data. The schematic shows a sequence of image processing steps that can be used to map how aging and dementia affect the cortex. The steps include aligning MRI data to a standard space, tissue classification, cortical pattern matching, as well as averaging and comparing local measures of cortical gray matter volumes across subjects. (These procedures are detailed in the main text). To help compare cortical features from subjects whose anatomy differs, individual gyral patterns are flattened and aligned with a group average gyral pattern (a to f). Group variability (g) and cortical asymmetry can also be computed. Correlations can be mapped between disease-related gray matter deficits and genetic risk factors. Maps may also be generated visualizing linkages between deficits and clinical symptoms, cognitive scores, and medication effects. The only steps here that are currently not automated are the tracing of sulci on the cortex. Some manual editing may also be required to assist algorithms that delete dura and scalp from images, especially if there is very little CSF in the diploic space.

Registration and Tissue Mapping

3D volumetric MRI scans are first rotated and scaled to match a standardized brain template in stereotaxic space. This template may either be an average intensity brain dataset constructed from a population of young normal subjects (Mazziotta et al. 2000 or one specially constructed to reflect the average anatomy of elderly subjects (e.g., Thompson et al. 2000c; Mega et al. 2000; Janke et al. 2001; see these papers for a discussion of *disease-specific* templates). Once aligned, a measure of the brain scaling imposed is retained as a covariate for statistical analysis. If a given subject has been scanned repeatedly, the same scaling is applied to both baseline and follow-up scans, to ensure that observed differences reflect true brain atrophy. A tissue classification algorithm then splits up the scan into regions representing gray matter, white matter, cerebrospinal fluid (CSF), and non-brain tissues. Stereotaxic maps of gray matter are retained.

Cortical Pattern Matching

MRI scans have sufficient resolution and tissue contrast, in principle, to track cortical gray matter loss in individual patients. Even so, extreme variability in gyral patterns confounds efforts 1) to compare this loss against a normative population and 2) to determine the average profile of tissue loss in a group. Cortical pattern matching methods (CPM; detailed further in Fig. 2) address these challenges. They encode both gyral patterning and gray matter variation. This encoding can substantially improve the statistical power to localize deficits. These cortical analyses tease apart the effects of gyral shape variation from gray matter change, and they can also be used to measure cortical asymmetries (Thompson et al. 2001e; Sowell et al. 2001). Briefly, a 3D geometric model of the cortical surface is extracted from the MRI scan and flattened to a 2D planar format (to avoid making cuts, a spherical topology can be retained; Fischl et al. 1999; Thompson et al. 1997a, b; 2002. A complex deformation, or warping transform, is then applied that aligns the sulcal anatomy of each subject with an average sulcal pattern derived for the group. To improve feature alignment across subjects, all sulci that occur consistently can be digitized (Hayashi et al. 2002), and used to constrain this transformation. As far as possible, this procedure adjusts for differences in cortical patterning and shape across subjects. Cortical measures can then be compared across subjects and groups. Sulcal landmarks are used as anchors, as homologous cortical regions are better aligned after matching sulci than by just averaging data at each point in stereotaxic space (see, e.g., functional MRI studies by Zeineh et al. 2001, 2003a, b; Rex et al. 2000; Rasser et al. 2003). Given that the deformation maps associate cortical locations with the same relation to the primary folding pattern across subjects, a local measurement of gray matter density is made in each subject and *averaged across equivalent cortical locations*. To quantify local gray matter, we use a measure termed *"gray matter density,"* used in many prior studies to compare the spatial distribution of gray matter across subjects. This measures the proportion of gray matter in a small region of fixed radius (15 mm) around each cortical point (Wright et al. 1995; Bullmore et al. 1999; Sowell et al. 1999, 2003; Ashburner and Friston 2000; Rombouts et al. 2000; Mummery et al. 2000; Thompson et al. 2001a,b; Good et al. 2001; Baron et al. 2001). Given the large anatomic variability in some cortical regions, high-dimensional elastic matching of cortical patterns (Thompson et al. 2000a, 2001f) is used to associate measures of gray matter density from homologous cortical regions first across time and then also across subjects (as shown in Fig. 2). One advantage of cortical matching is that it localizes deficits relative to gyral landmarks; it also averages data from corresponding gyri, which would be impossible if data were only linearly mapped

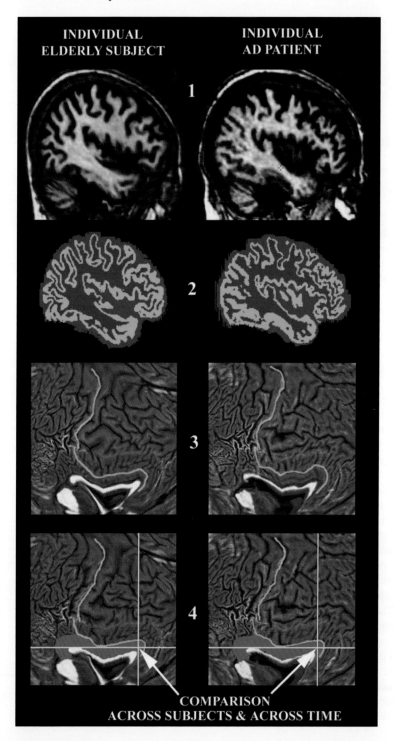

INDIVIDUAL ELDERLY SUBJECT

INDIVIDUAL AD PATIENT

1

2

3

4

COMPARISON
ACROSS SUBJECTS & ACROSS TIME

Fig. 2. Comparing gray matter across subjects. Gray matter is easier to compare across subjects if adjustments are first made for the gyral patterning differences across subjects. This adjustment can be made using cortical pattern matching (Thompson et al. 2000), which is illustrated here on sample brain MRI datasets from a healthy control subject (left column) and from a patient with Alzheimer's disease (right column). First, the MRI images (stage 1) have extracerebral tissues deleted from the scans and the individual pixels are classified as gray matter, white matter or CSF (shown here in green, red, and blue; stage 2). After flattening a 3D geometric model of the cortex (stage 3), features such as the central sulcus (light blue curve), and cingulate sulcus (green curve) may be reidentified (Hayashi et al. 2002). An elastic warp is applied (stage 4) moving these features, and entire gyral regions (pink), into the same reference position in "flat space" (cf. van Essen et al. 1997). After aligning sulcal patterns from all individual subjects, group comparisons can be made at each 2D pixel (yellow cross-hairs) that effectively compare gray matter measures across corresponding cortical regions. In this study, the cortical measure that is compared, across groups, and over time, is the amount of gray matter (stage 2) lying within 15 mm of each cortical point. The results of these statistical comparisons can then be plotted back onto an average 3D cortical model made for the group, and significant findings can be visualized as color-coded maps. Such algorithms bring gray matter maps from different subjects into a common anatomical reference space, overcoming individual differences in gyral patterns and shape by matching locations point-by-point throughout cortex. This enhances the precision of inter-subject statistical procedures to detect localized changes in gray matter.

◄————————————————————————————————

into stereotaxic space. Annualized 4D maps of gray matter loss rates within each subject are then elastically realigned for averaging and comparison across diagnostic groups (Fig. 1). The effects of age, gender, medication, disease and other measures on gray matter can be assessed at each cortical point.

Statistical Maps

An algorithm then fits a statistical model, such as the general linear model (GLM; Friston et al. 1995) to the data at each cortical location. This results in a variety of parameters that characterize how gray matter variation is linked with other variables. The significance of these links can be plotted as a significance map. A color code can highlight brain regions where linkages are found, allowing us to visualize the strength of these linkages. In addition, estimated parameters can be plotted, such as 1) the local rates of gray matter loss at each cortical location (e.g., as a percentage change per year), 2) regression parameters that identify disease effects, and even 3) nonlinearities in the rates of brain change over time (e.g., quadratic regression coefficients; Sowell et al. 2003). In principle, any statistical model can be fitted, including genetic models that estimate genetic or allelic influences on brain structure (Thompson et al. 2003d). Finally, permutation testing is typically used to ascribe an overall significance value for the observed map. This adjusts for the fact that multiple statistical tests are made when a whole map of statistics is visualized. Patients and controls are randomly assigned to groups, often many millions of times on a supercomputer. A null distribution is built to estimate the probability that the observed effects could have occurred by chance, and this is reported as a significance value for the overall map.

Gray Matter Deficits in Mild to Moderate AD

Our early AD work led to the first detailed maps of cortical gray matter loss in a diseased population (Fig. 3; Thompson *et al.* 2001b). High-resolution 3D MRI volumes were acquired from 26 subjects with mild to moderate AD (age: 75.8 ± 1.7 yrs.; MMSE score: 20.0 ± 0.9), and 20 normal elderly controls (72.4 ± 1.3 yrs.) matched for age, sex, handedness and educational level. In the AD cohort, average maps revealed complex profiles of gray matter loss, with severe reductions in gray matter (20-30% loss, $p<0.001$-0.0001) across the lateral temporal surfaces in the AD cohort. There was also a comparative sparing of superior postcentral and central gyri and the occipital poles (0%-5% loss; $p > 0.05$). At this stage, the pathologic burden of AD may be greater in terms of functional deficits, and in synaptic loss, in heteromodal cortex than in idiotypic cortex. This pattern is consistent with the preservation of sensorimotor and visual function at this stage of the disease, at the same time as perfusion and metabolic deficits pervade in higher order association cortices. Greatest gray matter loss in temporo-parietal cortex may underlie the prominent temporal-parietal hypometabolism found consistently at this stage of AD, often asymmetrically (with great impairments in the left hemisphere; Friedland and Luxenberg 1988; Johnson et al. 1998). In AD, relatively greater atrophy is often reported in temporal lobe relative to overall cerebral volume (Murphy et al. 1993). The early progression of AD pathology into parietal and frontal association cortices suggests a degeneration of synaptically linked cortical pathways, and this pattern correlates with symptoms of memory impairment, aphasia, apraxia, personality changes and spatial deficits (Roberts et al. 1993). Interestingly, gray matter loss at autopsy is predominantly cortical in Alzheimer's patients under 80 years of age (Hubbard and Anderson 1981), when volumes of subcortical nuclei are not significantly different between patients and controls (De La Monte 1989). Nonetheless, atrophy of the amygdala and basal nuclei (Cuénod et al. 1993) may ultimately be followed by alterations in thalamic nuclei (Jernigan et al. 1991), induced perhaps by degeneration of their cortical projection areas.

Beta-Amyloid Maps

There is also a remarkably strong spatial agreement between MRI-based maps of cortical atrophy, and post mortem maps of beta-amyloid deposition (Aβ; in Fig. 3, compare the MRI maps with Braak Stage B; Braak and Braak 1997). Beta-amyloid is an insoluble protein that is a key feature of Alzheimer pathology. The spatial congruence of these two maps supports the hypothesis that Aβ deposition may participate in the cascade of events that leads to regional gray matter atrophy and neuronal cell loss. In both maps, primary sensorimotor cortices are relatively spared until late in the disease, and the superior temporal gyrus is less affected than other temporal lobe gyri.

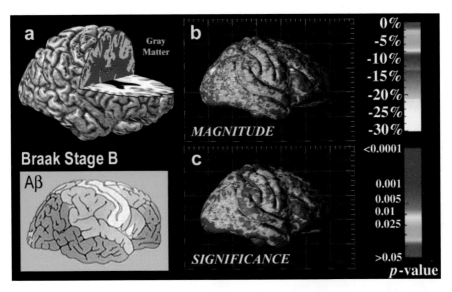

Fig. 3. Gray matter deficits in early AD. a) The local amount of cortical gray matter (shown in green) is compared across 26 patients with mild to moderate AD (age: 75.8±1.7 yrs.; MMSE score: 20.0±0.9) and 20 matched elderly controls (72.4±1.3 yrs.). At this stage of AD, there is a reduction in gray matter reaching 30% in the temporoparietal regions (b). c) A map of the statistical significance of these deficits. Intriguingly, the pattern of temporal lobe gray matter loss, seen with MRI, spatially matches the pattern of beta-amyloid (Aβ) deposition seen post mortem (Braak and Braak 1991, 1997; Braak et al. 2000). The **inset panel** (Braak Stage B) is adapted from data reported by Braak and Braak (1997). It shows regions with minimal (white), moderate (orange), and severe (red) beta amyloid deposition. Because amyloid deposition and gray matter loss may not be synchronized, these maps may represent different stages of AD; however, there is a clear spatial agreement in the severity of the deficits, between MRI and beta amyloid maps. Intriguingly, both maps indicated the relative sparing of primary sensorimotor regions (white in the amyloid map) and the superior temporal gyrus (blue in c) relative to other temporal lobe gyri. These overall MRI patterns have been replicated in independent studies by Baron et al. (2001), O'Brien et al. (2001), and Burton et al. (2002).

Transient Boundaries

In the statistical maps generated from CPM, anatomical divisions are resolved in temporal cortex, between severely and comparatively unaffected regions. These boundaries may only be transient, as ultimately the entire cortex is affected in AD. However, the cortical divisions appear not to be an artifact of the method. Gray matter variance maps reveal that they are not due to spatial differences in the statistical power to resolve group differences. For example, the cortical boundaries evident in the maps of group differences in gray matter density for AD delimit regions with opposite patterns of deficits in other disorders. In schizophrenia, for example, the most severely affected regions have an approximately opposite spatial pattern and timing to that shown here (Vidal et al, 2003; see Thompson et

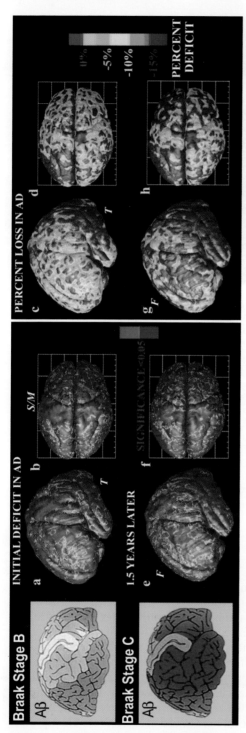

Fig. 4. Gray matter deficits sweep anteriorly in moderate AD. Deficits occurring during the development of AD are detected by comparing average profiles of gray matter between 12 AD patients (age: 68.4±1.9 yrs.) and 14 elderly matched controls (age: 71.4±0.9 yrs.). Patients and controls are subtracted at their first scan (when mean MMSE=18 for the patients; top row) and their follow-up scan 1.5 years later (mean MMSE=13; bottom row). The average percent loss in patients is shown in the right four panels, and the significance of this loss is shown in the left four panels. Although severe temporal lobe loss (T) and parietal loss have already occurred at baseline (top row), and subsequently continue, the frontal deficits (F) characteristic of late AD are not found until significant global cognitive decline has occurred (bottom row). A process of rapid attrition occurs over the 1.5 years after the baseline scan. Sensorimotor cortices are relatively spared at both disease stages (S/M). Regionally significant effects are coded red and assessed by permutation, which corrects for multiple comparisons. Note the agreement of these MRI-based changes, observed in living patients, with the progression of beta-amyloid (Aβ) pathology observed post mortem (Braak Stages B and C; left panels adapted from Braak and Braak, 1997).

al. 2002c, 2003c) for a comparison). After cortical pattern matching, sharp cortical boundaries often emerge in the population maps, allowing visualization of
divisions between severely and mildly affected brain regions (Fig. 3). Since gyral
pattern information is used when averaging anatomical models (Thompson et
al. 1997a, b), generic features of anatomy come into focus. On these geometric
models, statistics of group differences, or effects of covariates (age, sex, cognitive
scores), are defined. Differences can be visualized locally in the form of color-
coded statistical maps.

Video Maps of Disease Progression in AD

In a subsequent longitudinal study of an independent patient cohort from our
earlier cross sectional studies (Thompson et al. 2001b), we detected and mapped
a dynamically spreading wave of gray matter loss in the brains of patients with
AD (Thompson et al. 2003b). We analyzed 52 high-resolution MRI scans of 12
AD patients (age 68.4±1.9 years) and 14 elderly matched controls (age 71.4±0.9
years) scanned longitudinally (two scans; interscan interval 2.1±0.4 years). Novel
brain mapping methods allowed visualization of the loss pattern as it spread over
time from temporal and limbic cortices into frontal and occipital brain regions,
sparing sensorimotor cortices. The shifting deficits correlated extremely strongly
with progressively declining cognitive status ($p<0.0006$). As shown in Figure 4,
cortical atrophy occurred in a well-defined sequence as the disease progressed,
again mirroring the temporal sequence of $A\beta$ and NFT accumulation observed at
autopsy (Braak and Braak 1997). The trajectory of deficits also appeared to match
the sequence of metabolic decline typically observed with positron emission tomography (PET).

In the study mapping AD progression, advancing deficits were visualized as
dynamic video maps that change over time. Frontal regions, spared early in the
disease, showed pervasive deficits later (>15% loss). The maps distinguished different phases of AD and differentiated AD from normal aging. Local gray matter
loss rates (5.3±2.3% per year in AD versus 0.9±0.9% per year in controls) were
faster in the left hemisphere ($p<0.029$) than the right, at least at this stage of AD.
Transient barriers to disease progression appeared at limbic/frontal boundaries.
A frontal band (0-5% loss) was sharply delimited from the limbic and temporo-
parietal regions that showed severest deficits in AD (>15% loss). This pattern is
consistent with the hypothesis that AD pathology spreads centrifugally from lim-
bic/paralimbic to higher-order association cortices (Mesulam 2000). This degenerative sequence, observed as it developed in living patients, provided the first
quantitative, dynamic visualization of cortical atrophic rates in normal elderly
populations and in those with dementia. The time-course of these gray matter
losses, as they emerge over a period of cognitive decline lasting 1.5 years, is observed in a set of video sequences (see url, http://www.loni.ucla.edu/~thompson/
AD_4D/dynamic.html for several of these time-lapse movies).

100   Paul M. Thompson et al.

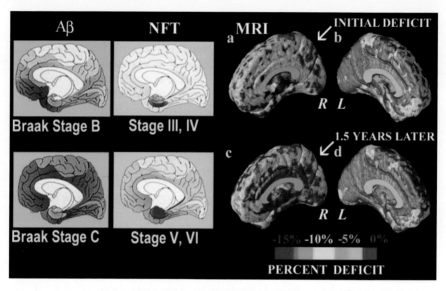

Fig. 5. Gray matter deficits spreading through the limbic system in moderate AD. Deficits occurring during the progression of AD are detected by comparing average profiles of gray matter between 12 AD patients (age: 68.4±1.9 yrs.) and 14 elderly matched controls (age: 71.4±0.9 yrs.). Patients and controls are subtracted at their first scan (when mean MMSE=18 for the patients (a and b) and their follow-up scan 1.5 years later (mean MMSE=13; c and d). Colors show the average percent loss of gray matter relative to the control average. Profound loss engulfs the left medial wall (>15%; b,d). On the right however, the deficits in temporo-parietal and entorhinal territory (a) spread forward into the cingulate 1.5 years later (c), after a 5 point drop in average MMSE. Note the prominent division between limbic and frontal zones, with different degrees of impairment (c). The corpus callosum is indicated in white; maps of gray matter change are not defined here, as it is a white matter commissure. MRI-based changes, observed in living patients, agree strongly with the spatial progression of beta-amyloid (Aβ) and neurofibrillary tangle (NFT) pathology observed post mortem (Braak Stages B,C and III to VI; left four panels adapted from Braak and Braak 1997). The deficit sequence also matches the trajectory of neurofibrillary tangle distribution observed post mortem in patients with increasing dementia severity at death (Braak and Braak 1997). Consistent with the deficit maps observed here, NFT accumulation is minimal in sensory and motor cortices, but occurs preferentially in entorhinal pyramidal cells, the limbic periallocortex (layers II/IV), the hippocampus/amygdala and subiculum, the basal forebrain cholinergic systems and subsequently in temporo-parietal and frontal association cortices (layers III/V; Pearson et al. 1985; Arnold et al. 1991). Neuropathologic studies also reveal that cortical layers III and V selectively lose large pyramidal neurons in association areas (Brun and Englund 1981; cf. Hyman et al. 1990).

Cognitive Linkage Maps

Ultimately, it is vital to understand how fine-scale volume changes on MRI relate to clinically meaningful endpoints (Kaye 2000). An important finding by Fox and associates (1999) was that the rate of hippocampal tissue degeneration in AD over time correlates with the rate of cognitive decline, reflected by worsening performance on the MMSE. In a recent 52-week clinical trial of milameline (a muscarinic receptor agonist), Jack et al. (2003) noted that hippocampal volume, measured with MRI, was a sensitive biomarker that tracked cognitive decline. Using statistical maps we have described, it is also possible to map cortical regions in which quantifiable variations in imaging biomarkers (here a local measure of cortical gray matter volume) are linked with declining cognitive function. To illustrate this approach, Figure 6 shows brain regions where cortical gray matter atrophy links with MMSE score in an AD population.

What is Gray Matter Atrophy?

Gray matter atrophy observed with MRI is linked with cognitive decline in AD and is attributable to several processes. In addition to overt neuronal loss, cell shrinkage, reduced dendritic extent, and synaptic loss occur in AD (see McEwen 1997 and Uylings and de Brabander 2002 for recent reviews). In healthy aging, age-related neuronal loss does not occur in most neocortical regions (Terry et al. 1987, 1991; Morrison and Hof 1997) and appears specific to the frontal cortex (de Brabander et al. 1998) and some hippocampal regions (e.g., CA1 and the subiculum; Simic et al. 1997; Peters et al. 1998). By contrast, marked neuronal loss occurs in early AD (Gomez-Isla et al. 1996), with severe early losses in layer II of the entorhinal cortex. Normal age-related cortical changes may reflect cell shrinkage (Shimada 1999), reduced dendritic length (Flood et al. 1987; Hanks and Flood 1991), and changes in perfusion, fat and water content and other chemical constituents (Weinberger and McClure 2002). Age-related dendritic reduction may be region- and lamina-specific (Uylings and Brabander 2002). Nakamura et al. (1984) found the greatest reductions in layer V pyramidal basal dendrites with normal aging; dentate granule cells also display significantly reduced apical dendritic length (>40% in the dentate gyrus; Hanks and Flood 1991). In summary, changes observed here in normal aging may primarily reflect cell shrinkage, reductions in dendritic extent, and synaptic loss; in AD, there is also substantial neuronal loss (Gomez-Isla et al. 1996).

Nonlinear Dynamics of Gray Matter Changes
Across the Human Life Span (n=176)

The quest for information on brain aging can also be advanced by collecting cortical brain maps over the entire human life span. The dynamics of brain change across the adult human life span are highly nonlinear (Jernigan et al. 1991; Bartzokis et al. 2001; Ge et al. 2002). To improve the statistical analysis of brain change, we recently developed a set of statistical mapping approaches to estimate nonlinear (quadratic) effects of aging on brain structure.

In a recent study (Sowell et al. 2003; Fig. 7), we used MRI and cortical matching algorithms to map gray matter density (GMD) in 176 normal individuals aged 7 to 87 years. GMD declined nonlinearly with age, most quickly between ages 7 and 60, over dorsal frontal and parietal association cortices on both the lateral and

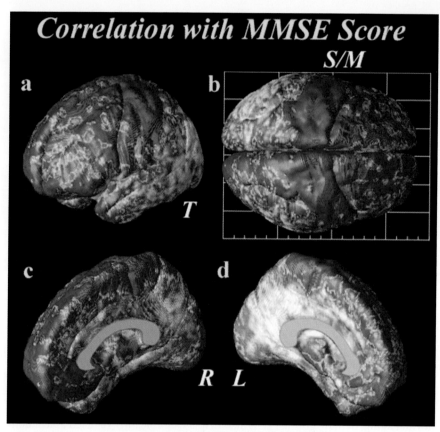

Fig. 6. Maps correlating brain structure with cognitive decline. In addition to providing a sensitive index of how disease impacts the cortex, it is vital to verify that structural measures are in fact linked with cognitive decline (Kaye et al. 1999). This map shows brain regions where a lower MMSE score is linked with reduced gray matter volumes in a cohort of serially scanned subjects with AD (Thompson et al. 2003b). Ongoing work by our group and others (Janke et al. 2001; Fox et al. 2001) has identified several MRI-based biological markers that are tightly linked with cognitive decline. Using a population database, it is also possible to search for (and subsequently validate) neuroimaging variations that link with specific clinical stages or risk factors. This can be achieved by correlating maps of anatomical deficits with a variety of neurocognitive test data, IQ measures and even genetic information (Thompson et al. 2001a; cf. Hyman et al. 1996). Permutation testing can then be employed to safeguard against finding "false positive" (i.e., spurious) associations (Bullmore et al. 1999; Thompson et al. 2001a; 2003a).

interhemispheric surfaces. Age effects were inverted in the left posterior temporal region, where GMD gain continued up to age 30, and then rapidly declined. This was the first study to differentiate the trajectory of maturational and aging effects as they vary over the cortex. Visual, auditory and limbic cortices, which myelinate early, showed a more linear pattern of aging than the frontal and parietal neocortices, which continue myelination into adulthood. Posterior temporal

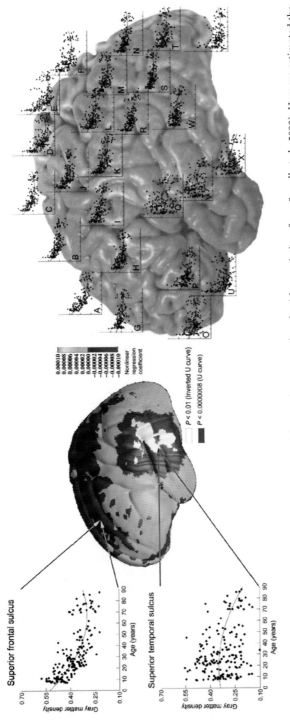

Fig. 7. Mapping nonlinear brain change across the human life span (Data reproduced, with permission, from Sowell et al., 2003). Here we estimated the trajectory of cortical gray matter loss across the human life span. Gray matter density was measured in a cohort of 176 normal subjects. After cortical pattern matching was used to associate data from corresponding cortical regions, we developed software to fit a general, nonlinear statistical model to the gray matter data from the population. This revealed significant nonlinear (quadratic) effects of time on brain structure. The techniques allow trajectories of brain change to be mapped. Based on these algorithms, it is possible to compare these trajectories with those found in dementia populations and those at risk. To accommodate serial MRI data, this analysis requires the development of nonlinear mixed models on manifolds (Thompson et al. 2003b). This difficult mathematical area is likely to have extremely high power to resolve cohort and treatment effects, even greater than that already demonstrated for mapping brain change in healthy controls.

cortices, primarily in the left hemisphere, which typically support language functions, have a more protracted course of maturation than any other cortical region. Overall, these observations support the hypothesis (Braak and Braak 1997) that the atrophic trajectory in AD is somewhat the reverse of the sequence in which cortical areas are myelinated during development. For example, primary sensory regions myelinate first and degenerate last, whereas temporal regions mature last but degenerate first in AD. We are currently testing whether this palindromic sequence is observed when cortical changes are observed more locally in the cortex. The selective vulnerability of specific cortical systems in AD may relate to differences in cellular maturational rates and/or plasticity (Mesulam 2000).

Dynamic Maps of Brain Change

Statistical brain maps from large populations (Fig. 7) are likely to help assess how different drug treatments affect the time course of aging and dementia. In developing dynamic atlases for clinical applications, there is a particular interest in modeling atrophic processes that speed up or slow down. Diseases may accelerate or their rate of progression may be slowed down by therapy. If individuals are scanned more than twice over large time spans (e.g., Fox et al. 2001; Janke et al. 2001), brain change can be modeled more accurately. To compare atrophic processes in different groups of subjects, nonlinear mixed models can be used (Giedd et al. 1999; Toga and Thompson 2003a, b) to analyze the registered degenerative profiles. For the ith individual's jth measure we have:

$$Y_{ij} = f(\text{Age}_{ij}, \underline{\beta}) + \varepsilon_{ij}$$

Here Y_{ij} signifies the outcome measure at a voxel or surface point, such as growth or tissue loss, $f()$ denotes a constant, linear, quadratic, cubic, or other function of the individual's age for that scan, and $\underline{\beta}$ denotes the regression/ANOVA coefficients to be estimated. In models whose fit is confirmed as significant, e.g., by permutation, loadings on nonlinear parameters may be visualized as attribute maps $\beta(\mathbf{x})$. This reveals the topography of accelerated or decelerated brain change (Thompson et al. 2001b). The result is a formal approach to assess whether, and where, brain change is speeding up or slowing down, a key feature in medication studies.

In this statistical model, Age (Age_{ij}) may be replaced by time from the onset of disease or medication. This flexibility in parameterizing the time axis allows one to temporally register dynamic patterns using criteria that are expected to bring into line temporal features of interest that appear systematically in a group (Janke et al. 2001). For example, the independent variable could be a cognitive score such as Mini-Mental status (Janke et al. 2001), which declines over time in AD. Parameterization of dynamic effects using measures other than time (e.g., clinical status) also provides a mechanism to align new patients' time series with a dynamic atlas (Janke et al. 2001), potentially still further increasing the power to reveal systematic effects.

Conclusion

As a whole, the mapping methods described here differ substantially from volumetric measures of anatomy used in conventional studies (see Thompson et al. 2003a,c for a comparison). By contrast, brain mapping algorithms use longitudinal MRI data to create spatially detailed maps of brain change, allowing visualization of rates and profiles of tissue loss throughout the whole brain. Computational atlases can store these maps from large patient cohorts, including those at genetic risk. They can uncover nonlinear brain changes over the human life span and chart the path of cortical change in dementia. There are two urgent applications of these atlasing methods. The first is to map therapeutic effects in drug trials that aim to slow disease progression. Dynamic maps have potential as a surrogate outcome measure for disease stabilization therapies, providing regional anatomic localization of any beneficial effects. Any improvement in the set of neuroimaging biomarkers will make it considerably easier to monitor the proactive benefits of treatment before the disease progresses to the point of disrupting global cognitive functions. Secondly, there is interest in developing neuroimaging markers that can predict early transition to dementia in otherwise healthy elderly subjects with mild cognitive impairment (MCI; Kaye et al. 1997, 1999; Jack et al. 1999; Convit et al. 2000; Du et al. 2001). Recently, an analysis of pre-symptomatic scans suggested that atrophic rates accelerate starting five years before diagnosis (Fox et al. 2001). This research is highly significant because, in the absence of a neuroimaging marker, by the time preclinical AD has progressed to dementia, widespread irreversible neuronal loss has occurred. The structural and metabolic maps, along with measures of genetic risk and abnormalities in specific neuropsychological tests, now provide key quantitative predictors to monitor brain degeneration and gauge how well it is decelerated or delayed in clinical trials.

Acknowledgments

This work was supported by research grants from the National Center for Research Resources (P41 RR13642 and R21 RR19771), the National Library of Medicine (LM/MH05639), National Institute of Neurological Disorders and Stroke and the National Institute of Mental Health (NINDS/NIMH NS38753 and NIMH MH01733), the National Institute for Biomedical Imaging and Bioengineering (R21 EB001561), GlaxoSmithKline Pharmaceuticals UK, and by a Human Brain Project grant to the International Consortium for Brain Mapping, funded jointly by NIMH and NIDA (P20 MH/DA52176). We also appreciate the support of Jacqueline Mervaillie, Yves Christen, Brad Hyman, and the members of the IPSEN Foundation for hosting the Colloque Médecine et Recherche, at which these findings were reported.

References

Arnold SE, Hyman BT, Flory J, Damasio AR, Van Hoesen GW (1991) The topographical and neuroanatomical distribution of neurofibrillary tangles and neuritic plaques in the cerebral cortex of patients with Alzheimer's disease. Cereb Cortex 1:103–116

Ashburner J, Friston KJ (2000) Voxel-based morphometry--the methods. Neuroimage 11, 6:805–821

Ashburner J, Csernansky J, Davatzikos C, Fox NC, Frisoni G, Thompson PM (2003) Computer-assisted imaging to assess brain structure in healthy and diseased brains. Lancet Neurol 2:79–88

Baron JC, Chetelat G, Desgranges B, Perchey G, Landeau B, de la Sayette V, Eustache F (2001) In vivo mapping of gray matter loss with voxel-based morphometry in mild Alzheimer's disease. Neuroimage 14: 298–309

Bartzokis G, Beckson M, Lu PH, Nuechterlein KH, Edwards N, Mintz J (2001) Age-related changes in frontal and temporal lobe volumes in men: a magnetic resonance imaging study. Arch Gen Psychiatry 58: 461–465

Black SE (1999) The search for diagnostic and progression markers in AD: so near but still too far? Neurology 52:1533–1534

Braak H, Braak E (1997) Staging of Alzheimer-related cortical destruction. Int Psychogeriatr 9 Suppl 1:257-261; discussion 269–272

Bradley KM, Bydder GM, Budge MM, Hajnal JV, White SJ, Ripley BD, Smith AD (2002). Serial brain MRI at 3–6 month intervals as a surrogate marker for Alzheimer's disease. Br J Radiol 75:506–13

Brun A, Englund E (1981) Regional pattern of degeneration in Alzheimer's disease: Neuronal loss and histopathologic grading, Histopathology 5:549–564

Bullmore ET, Suckling J, Overmeyer S, Rabe-Hesketh S, Taylor E, Brammer MJ (1999) Global, voxel, and cluster tests, by theory and permutation, for a difference between two groups of structural MR images of the brain. IEEE Trans Med Imag 18:32–42

Burton EJ, Karas G, Paling SM, Barber R, Williams ED, Ballard CG, McKeith IG, Scheltens P, Barkhof F, O'Brien JT (2002) Patterns of cerebral atrophy in dementia with Lewy bodies using voxel-based morphometry. Neuroimage. 17:618–630

Chan D, Fox NC, Jenkins R, Scahill RI, Crum WR, Rossor MN (2001) Rates of global and regional cerebral atrophy in AD and frontotemporal dementia. Neurology 57: 1756–1763

Chetelat G, Baron JC (2003). Early diagnosis of Alzheimer's disease: contribution of structural neuroimaging. Neuroimage 18:525–541

Convit A, de Asis J, de Leon MJ, Tarshish CY, De Santi S, Rusinek H (2000) Atrophy of the medial occipitotemporal, inferior, and middle temporal gyri in non-demented elderly predict decline to Alzheimer's disease. Neurobiol Aging 21: 19–26

Crum WR, Scahill RI, Fox NC (2001) Automated hippocampal segmentation by regional fluid registration of serial MRI: validation and application in Alzheimer's disease. Neuroimage 13: 847-855

Csernansky JG, Wang L, Joshi S, Miller JP, Gado M, Kido D, McKeel D, Morris JC, Miller MI (2000) Early DAT is distinguished from aging by high-dimensional mapping of the hippocampus. Dementia of the Alzheimer type. Neurology 55:1636–1643

Cuénod CA, Denys A, Michot JL, Jehenson P, Forette F, Kaplan D, Syrota A, Boller F (1993) Amygdala atrophy in Alzheimer's disease. An in vivo magnetic resonance imaging study. Arch Neurol 50:941–945

Davatzikos C, Genc A, Xu D, Resnick SM (2001) Voxel-based morphometry using the RAVENS maps: methods and validation using simulated longitudinal atrophy. Neuroimage. 14:1361–1369

Davatzikos C, Resnick SM (2002) Degenerative age changes in white matter connectivity visualized in vivo using magnetic resonance imaging. Cereb Cortex, 12:767–771

de Brabander JM, Kramers RJ, Uylings HB (1998) Layer-specific dendritic regression of pyramidal cells with aging in the human prefrontal cortex. Eur J Neurosci 10:1261–1269

De La Monte SM (1989) Quantitation of cerebral atrophy in preclinical and end-stage Alzheimer's disease. Ann Neurol 25:450–459

De Leon MJ, George AE, Golomb J, Tarshish C, Convit A, Kluger A, De Santi S, McRae T, Ferris SH, Reisberg B, Ince C, Rusinek H, Bobinski M, Quinn B, Miller DC, Wisniewski HM (1997) Frequency of hippocampal formation atrophy in normal aging and Alzheimer's disease. Neurobiol Aging 18:1–11

Delacourte A, David JP, Sergeant N, Buee L, Wattez A, Vermersch P, Ghozali F, Fallet-Bianco C, Pasquier F, Lebert F, Petit H, Di Menza C (1999) The biochemical pathway of neurofibrillary degeneration in aging and Alzheimer's disease. Neurology 52:1158–1165

Dickerson BC, Goncharova I, Sullivan MP, Forchetti C, Wilson RS, Bennett DA, Beckett LA, de-Toledo-Morrell L (2001) MRI-derived entorhinal and hippocampal atrophy in incipient and very mild Alzheimer's disease. Neurobiol Aging 22:747–754

Du AT, Schuff N, Amend D, Laakso MP, Hsu YY, Jagust WJ, Yaffe K, Kramer JH, Reed B, Norman D, Chui HC, Weiner MW (2001) Magnetic resonance imaging of the entorhinal cortex and hippocampus in mild cognitive impairment and Alzheimer's disease. J Neurol Neurosurg Psychiat 71: 441–447

Fischl B, Sereno MI, Tootell RBH, Dale AM (1999) High-resolution inter-subject averaging and a coordinate system for the cortical surface. Human Brain Mapp 8:272–84

Flood DG, Buell SJ, Horwitz GJ, Coleman PD (1987) Dendritic extent in human dentate gyrus granule cells in normal aging and senile dementia. Brain Res 402:205–216

Folstein MF, Folstein SE, McHugh PR (1975) 'Mini mental state': a practical method of grading the cognitive state of patients for the clinician. J Psychiat Res 12:189–198

Forette F, Seux ML, Staessen JA, Thijs L, Babarskiene MR, Babeanu S, Bossini A, Fagard R, Gil-Extremera B, Laks T, Kobalava Z, Sarti C, Tuomilehto J, Vanhanen H, Webster J, Yodfat Y, Birkenhager WH. (2002) The prevention of dementia with antihypertensive treatment: new evidence from the systolic hypertension in Europe (syst-eur) study. Arch Intern Med 162:2046–2052

Fox NC, Freeborough PA (1997) Brain atrophy progression measured from registered serial MRI: validation and application to Alzheimer's disease. J Magn Reson Imag 7: 1069–1075

Fox NC, Freeborough PA, Rossor MN (1996) Visualisation and quantification of rates of atrophy in Alzheimer's disease. Lancet 348: 94–97

Fox NC, Cousens S, Scahill R, Harvey RJ, Rossor MN (2000) Using serial registered brain magnetic resonance imaging to measure disease progression in Alzheimer disease: power calculations and estimates of sample size to detect treatment effects. Arch Neurol 57: 339–344

Fox NC, Crum WR, Scahill RI, Stevens JM, Janssen JC, Rossor MN (2001) Imaging of onset and progression of Alzheimer's disease with voxel-compression mapping of serial magnetic resonance images. Lancet 358: 201–205

Friedland RP, Luxenberg J (1988) Neuroimaging and dementia. In: Theodore WH (ed) Clinical neuroimaging: frontiers in clinical neuroscience. Vol. 4. New York, Allan Liss, pp 139–163

Frisoni GB, Laakso MP, Beltramello A, Geroldi C, Bianchetti A, Soininen H, Trabucchi M (1999) Hippocampal and entorhinal cortex atrophy in frontotemporal dementia and Alzheimer's disease. Neurology 52: 91–100

Friston KJ, Holmes AP, Worsley KJ, Poline JP, Frith CD, Frackowiak RSJ (1995). Statistical parametric maps in functional imaging: a general linear approach. Human Brain Mapp 2:189–210

Ge Y, Grossman RI, Babb JS, Rabin ML, Mannon LJ, Kolson DL (2002) Age-related total gray matter and white matter changes in normal adult brain. part II: quantitative magnetization transfer ratio histogram analysis. Am J Neuroradiol 23:1334–1341

Giedd JN, Blumenthal J, Jeffries NO, Castellanos FX, Liu H, Zijdenbos A, Paus T, Evans AC, Rapoport JL (1999) Brain development during childhood and adolescence: a longitudinal MRI study. Nature Neurosci 2:861–863

Gomez-Isla T, Price JL, McKeel DW Jr, Morris JC, Growdon JH, Hyman BT (1996) Profound loss of layer II entorhinal cortex neurons occurs in very mild Alzheimer's disease. J Neurosci 16:4491–4500

Good CD, Johnsrude IS, Ashburner J, Henson RN, Friston KJ, Frackowiak RSJ (2001) A voxel-based morphometric study of ageing in 465 normal adult human brains. Neuroimage 14:21–36

Grenander U, Miller MI (1998) Computational anatomy: an emerging discipline. Quart Appl Math 4: 617–694

Grundman M, Sencakova D, Jack CR Jr, Petersen RC, Kim HT, Schultz A, Weiner MF, DeCarli C, DeKosky ST, van Dyck C, Thomas RG, Thal LJ (2002) Alzheimer's Disease Cooperative Study (2002). Brain MRI hippocampal volume and prediction of clinical status in a mild cognitive impairment trial. J Mol Neurosci 19:23–27

Haller JW, Banerjee A, Christensen GE, Gado M, Joshi S, Miller MI, Sheline Y, Vannier MW, Csernansky JG (1997) Three-dimensional hippocampal MR morphometry with high-dimensional transformation of a neuroanatomic atlas. Radiology 202:504–510

Hanks SD, Flood DG (1991) Region-specific stability of dendritic extent in normal human aging and regression in Alzheimer's disease. I. CA1 of hippocampus. Brain Res 540:63–82

Hayashi KM, Thompson PM, Mega MS, Zoumalan CI, Dittmer S (2002) Medial hemispheric surface gyral pattern delineation in 3D: surface curve protocol. Available via Internet: http://www.loni.ucla.edu/~khayashi/Public/medial_surface/

Hubbard BM, Anderson JM (1981) A quantitative study of cerebral atrophy in old age and senile dementia. J Neurol Sci 50:135–145

Hulstaert F, Blennow K, Ivanoiu A, Schoonderwaldt HC, Riemenschneider M, De Deyn PP, Bancher C, Cras P, Wiltfang J, Mehta PD, Iqbal K, Pottel H, Vanmechelen E, Vanderstichele H (1999) Improved discrimination of AD patients using beta-amyloid (1–42) and tau levels in CSF. Neurology 52:1555–1562

Hyman BT, Van Hoesen GW, Damasio AR (1990) Memory-related neural systems in Alzheimer's disease: an anatomic study. Neurology 40:1721-1730

Hyman BT, Gomez-Isla T, Rebeck GW, Briggs M, Chung H, West HL, Greenberg S, Mui S, Nichols S, Wallace R, Growdon JH (1996) Epidemiological, clinical, and neuropathological study of apolipoprotein E genotype in Alzheimer's disease. Ann NY Acad Sci 802:1–5

Jack CR Jr, Petersen RC, O'Brien PC, Tangalos EG (1992) MR-based hippocampal volumetry in the diagnosis of Alzheimer's disease. Neurology 42: 183–138

Jack CR Jr, Petersen RC, Xu YC, Waring SC, O'Brien PC, Tangalos EG, Smith GE, Ivnik RJ, Kokmen E (1997) Medial temporal atrophy on MRI in normal aging and very mild Alzheimer's disease. Neurology 49:786–794

Jack CR Jr, Petersen RC, Xu Y, O'Brien PC, Smith GE, Ivnik RJ, Tangalos EG, Kokmen E (1998) Rate of medial temporal lobe atrophy in typical aging and Alzheimer's disease. Neurology 51:993–999

Jack CR Jr, Petersen RC, Xu YC, O'Brien PC, Smith GE, Ivnik RJ, Boeve BF, Waring SC, Tangalos EG, Kokmen E (1999) Prediction of AD with MRI-based hippocampal volume in mild cognitive impairment. Neurology 52: 1397–1403

Jack CR Jr, Petersen RC, Xu Y, O'Brien PC, Smith GE, Ivnik RJ, Boeve BF, Tangalos EG, Kokmen E (2000) Rates of hippocampal atrophy correlate with change in clinical status in aging and AD. Neurology 55:484–489

Jack CR Jr, Slomkowski M, Gracon S, Hoover TM, Felmlee JP, Stewart K, Xu Y, Shiung M, O'Brien PC, Cha R, Knopman D, Petersen RC (2003) MRI as a biomarker of disease progression in a therapeutic trial of milameline for AD. Neurology 60:253–260

Janke AL, Zubicaray GD, Rose SE, Griffin M, Chalk JB, Galloway GJ (2001) 4D deformation modeling of cortical disease progression in Alzheimer's dementia. Magn Reson Med 46: 661–666

Jernigan TL, Archibald SL, Berhow MT, Sowell ER, Foster DS, Hesselink JR (1991) Cerebral structure on MRI, Part II: specific changes in Alzheimer's and Huntington's diseases. Biol Psychiat 29:68–81

Jobst KA, Smith AD, Szatmari M, Molyneux A, Esiri ME, King E, Smith A, Jaskowski A, McDonald B, Wald N (1992) Detection in life of confirmed Alzheimer's disease using a simple measurement of medial temporal lobe atrophy by computed tomography. Lancet 340:1179–1183

Jobst KA, Smith AD, Szatmari M, Esiri MM, Jaskowski A, Hindley N, McDonald B, Molyneux AJ (1994) Rapidly progressing atrophy of medial temporal lobe in Alzheimer's disease. Lancet 343:829–830

Johnson KA, Jones K, Holman BL, Becker JA, Spiers PA, Satlin A, Albert MS (1998) Preclinical prediction of Alzheimer's disease using SPECT. Neurology 50:1563–1571

Kaye JA (2000) Methods for discerning disease-modifying effects in Alzheimer disease treatment trials. Arch Neurol 57:312–314

Kaye J, Moore M, Kerr D, Quinn J, Camicioli R, Howieson D, Payami H, Sexton G (1999) The rate of brain volume loss accelerates as Alzheimer's disease progresses from a presymptomatic phase to frank dementia. Neurology 52:A569–A570

Kaye JA, Swihart T, Howieson D, Dame A, Moore MM, Karnos T, Camicioli R, Ball M, Oken B, Sexton G (1997) Volume loss of the hippocampus and temporal lobe in healthy elderly persons destined to develop dementia. Neurology 48:1297–1304

Laakso MP, Frisoni GB, Kononen M, Mikkonen M, Beltramello A, Geroldi C, Bianchetti A, Trabucchi M, Soininen H, Aronen HJ (2000a) Hippocampus and entorhinal cortex in frontotemporal dementia and Alzheimer's disease: a morphometric MRI study. Biol Psychiat 47:1056–1063

Laakso MP, Lehtovirta M, Partanen K, Riekkinen PJ, Soininen H (2000b) Hippocampus in AD: a 3-year follow-up MRI study. Biol Psychiat 47:557–561

Malmgren R (2000) Epidemiology of aging. In: Coffey CE, Cummings JL (eds) Textbook of geriatric neuropsychiatry. Washington, D.C., American Psychiatric Press, Inc., pp. 17–31

Mazziotta JC, Toga AW, Evans AC, Fox P, Lancaster J (1995) A probabilistic atlas of the human brain: theory and rationale for its development. NeuroImage 2: 89–101

Mazziotta JC, Toga AW, Evans AC, Fox PT, Lancaster J, Zilles K, Woods RP, Paus T, Simpson G, Pike B, Holmes CJ, Collins DL, Thompson PM, MacDonald D, Schormann T, Amunts K, Palomero-Gallagher N, Parsons L, Narr KL, Kabani N, Le Goualher G, Boomsma D, Cannon T, Kawashima R, Mazoyer B (2000) A probabilistic atlas and reference system for the human brain. Invited Paper. J Roy Soc 356:1293–1322

McEwen BS (1997) Possible mechanisms for atrophy of the human hippocampus. Mol Psychiat 2:255–262

Mega MS, Chen S, Thompson PM, Woods RP, Karaca TJ, Tiwari A, Vinters H, Small GW, Toga AW (1997) Mapping pathology to metabolism: coregistration of stained whole brain sections to PET in Alzheimer's disease. NeuroImage 5:147–153

Mega MS, Chu T, Mazziotta JC, Trivedi KH, Thompson PM, Shah A, Cole G, Frautschy SA, Toga AW (1999) Mapping biochemistry to metabolism: FDG-PET and beta-amyloid burden in Alzheimer's disease. NeuroReport 10:2911–2917

Mega MS, Thompson PM, Toga AW, Cummings JL (2000) Brain mapping in dementia, book chapter. In: Toga AW, Mazziotta JC (eds.) Brain mapping: the disorders. Academic Press pp 218–234

Meltzer CC, Frost JJ (1994) Partial volume correction in emission-computed tomography: focus on Alzheimer disease. In: Thatcher RW, Hallett M, Zeffiro T, John ER, Huerta M (eds) Functional neuroimaging. San Diego, Academic Press, pp. 163–170

Mesulam MM (2000) A plasticity-based theory of the pathogenesis of Alzheimer's disease. Ann NY Acad Sci 924:42–52

Miller MI, Trouve A, Younes L (2002) On the metrics and Euler-Lagrange equations of computational anatomy. Annu Rev Biomed Eng. 4:375–405

Morrison JH, Hof PR (1997) Life and death of neurons in the aging brain. Science 278:412–419

Mummery CJ, Patterson K, Price CJ, Ashburner J, Frackowiak RS, Hodges JR (2000) A voxel-based morphometry study of semantic dementia: relationship between temporal lobe atrophy and semantic memory. Ann Neurol 47:36–45

Murphy DGM, DeCarli CD, Daly E, Gillette JA, McIntosh AR, Haxby JV, Teichberg D, Schapiro MB, Rapoport SI, Horwitz B (1993) Volumetric magnetic resonance imaging in men with dementia of the Alzheimer type: correlations with disease severity. Biol Psychiat 34:612–621

Nakamura S, Koshimura K, Kato T, Yamao S, Iijima S, Nagata H, Miyata S, Fujiyoshi K, Okamoto K, Suga H, Kameyama M (1984) Neurotransmitters in dementia. Clin Ther. 7 Spec No:18–34

O'Brien JT, Paling S, Barber R, Williams ED, Ballard C, McKeith IG, Gholkar A, Crum WR, Rossor MN, Fox NC (2001) Progressive brain atrophy on serial MRI in dementia with Lewy bodies, AD, and vascular dementia. Neurology 56:1386–1388

Ohm TG, Muller H, Braak H, Bohl J (1995) Close-meshed prevalence rates of different stages as a tool to uncover the rate of Alzheimer's disease-related neurofibrillary changes. Neuroscience 64:209–217

Pearson RCA, Esiri MM, Hiorns RW, Wilcock GK, Powell TPS (1985) Anatomical correlates of the distribution of the pathological changes in the neocortex in Alzheimer's disease. Proc Natl Acad Sci USA 82:4531–4534

Peters A, Morrison JH, Rosene DL, Hyman BT (1998) Feature article: are neurons lost from the primate cerebral cortex during normal aging? Cereb Cortex 8:295-300

Price JL, Morris JC (1999) Tangles and plaques in nondemented aging and "preclinical" Alzheimer's disease Ann Neurol 45: 358-368

Price JL, Ko AI, Wade MJ, Tsou SK, McKeel DW, Morris JC (2001) Neuron number in the entorhinal cortex and CA1 in preclinical Alzheimer disease. Arch Neurol 58:1395-1402

Rasser PE, Johnston P, Lagopoulos J, Ward PB, Schall U, Thienel R, Bender S, Thompson PM (2003) Analysis of fMRI BOLD activation during the Tower of London Task using Cortical Pattern Matching. International Congress for Schizophrenia Research (ICSR), Colorado Springs, Colorado, March 29-April 2, 2003

Reiman EM, Caselli RJ, Chen K, Alexander GE, Bandy D, Frost J (2001) Declining brain activity in cognitively normal apolipoprotein E epsilon 4 heterozygotes: A foundation for using positron emission tomography to efficiently test treatments to prevent Alzheimer's disease. Proc Natl Acad Sci USA 98:3334-3339

Resnick SM, Goldszal AF, Davatzikos C, Golski, Kraut MA, Metter EJ, Bryan RN, Zonderman AB (2000) One-year age changes in MRI brain volumes in older adults. Cereb Cortex 10: 464-472

Rex DE, Pouratian N, Thompson PM, Cunanan CC, Sicotte NL, Collins RC, Toga AW (2000) Cortical surface warping applied to group analysis of fMRI of tongue movement in the left hemisphere. [abstract] Proc Soc Neurosci 26:2102

Roberts GW, Nash M, Ince PG, Royston MC, Gentleman SM (1993) On the origin of Alzheimer's disease: a hypothesis. Neuroreport 4:7-9

Rombouts SA, Barkhof F, Witter MP, Scheltens P (2000) Unbiased whole-brain analysis of gray matter loss in Alzheimer's disease. Neurosci Lett 285:231-233

Rosen HJ, Gorno-Tempini ML, Goldman WP, Perry RJ, Schuff N, Weiner M, Feiwell R, Kramer JH, Miller BL (2002) Patterns of brain atrophy in frontotemporal dementia and semantic dementia. Neurology 58: 198-208

Rossor MN, Fox NC, Freeborough PA, Roques PK (1997) Slowing the progression of Alzheimer disease: monitoring progression. Alzheimer Dis Assoc Disord 11 Suppl 5:S6-9

Scahill RI, Schott JM, Stevens JM, Rossor MN, Fox NC (2002) Mapping the evolution of regional atrophy in Alzheimer's disease: unbiased analysis of fluid-registered serial MRI. Proc Natl Acad Sci USA 99:4703-4707

Scheltens P, Fox N, Barkhof F, De Carli C (2002) Structural magnetic resonance imaging in the practical assessment of dementia: beyond exclusion. Lancet Neurol 1: 13-21

Shimada A (1999) Age-dependent cerebral atrophy and cognitive dysfunction in SAMP10 mice. Neurobiol Aging 20:125-136

Simic G, Kostovic I, Winblad B, Bogdanovic N (1997) Volume and number of neurons of the human hippocampal formation in normal aging and Alzheimer's disease. J Comp Neurol 379:482-494

Smith SM, De Stefano N, Jenkinson M, Matthews PM (2002) Measurement of brain change over time, FMRIB Technical Report TR00SMS1 http://www.fmrib.ox.ac.uk/analysis/research/siena/siena/siena.html

Sowell ER, Thompson PM, Holmes CJ, Jernigan TL, Toga AW (1999) Progression of structural changes in the human brain during the first three decades of life: in vivo evidence for post-adolescent frontal and striatal maturation, Nature Neurosci 2:859-861

Sowell ER, Thompson PM, Tessner KD, Toga AW (2001) Accelerated Brain Growth and Cortical Gray Matter Thinning are Inversely Related during Post-Adolescent Frontal Lobe Maturation. J Neurosci 21:8819-8829

Sowell ER, Thompson PM, Mattson SN, Tessner KD, Jernigan TL, Riley EP, Toga AW (2002) Regional brain shape abnormalities persist into adolescence after heavy prenatal alcohol exposure. Cereb Cortex 12:856-865

Sowell ER, Peterson B, Thompson PM, Henkenius A, Welcome SE, Toga AW, (2003) Mapping age related cortical changes across the human life span. Nature Neurosci 6:309-315

Studholme C, Cardenas V, Schuff N, Rosen H, Miller B, Weiner MW (2001) Detecting spatially consistent structural differences in Alzheimer's and fronto temporal dementia using deformation morphometry. MICCAI 41-48

Terry RD, DeTeresa R, Hansen LA (1987) Neocortical cell counts in normal human adult aging. Ann Neurol 21:530–539

Terry RD, Masliah E, Salmon DP, Butters N, DeTeresa R, Hill R, Hansen LA, Katzman R (1991) Physical basis of cognitive alterations in Alzheimer's disease: synapse loss is the major correlate of cognitive impairment. Ann Neurol 30:572–580

Thal DR, Rub U, Orantes M, Braak H (2002) Phases of A beta-deposition in the human brain and its relevance for the development of AD. Neurology 58:1791–1800

Thompson PM, Toga AW (1996) A surface-based technique for warping 3-dimensional images of the brain. IEEE Trans Med Imag 15:402–417

Thompson PM, Toga AW (1998) Anatomically-driven strategies for high-dimensional brain image warping and pathology detection. In: Toga AW (Ed) Brain warping. Academic Press, San Diego pp. 311–336

Thompson PM, Toga AW (2000) Elastic image registration and pathology detection. In: Bankman I, Rangayyan R, Evans AC, Woods RP, Fishman E, Huang HK (eds) Handbook of medical image processing. Academic Press

Thompson PM, Toga AW (2002) A framework for computational anatomy. Invited Paper. Comput Visual Sci 5:1–12

Thompson PM, Toga AW (2003) Cortical diseases and cortical localization. Nature Encycl Life Sci, in press

Thompson PM, Schwartz C, Lin RT, Khan AA, Toga AW (1996) 3D statistical analysis of sulcal variability in the human brain. J Neurosci 16:4261–4274

Thompson PM, MacDonald D, Mega MS, Holmes CJ, Evans AC, Toga AW (1997a) Detection and mapping of abnormal brain structure with a probabilistic atlas of cortical surfaces. J Comp Assist Tomograph 21:567–581

Thompson PM, Toga AW (1997b) Detection, visualization and animation of abnormal anatomic structure with a deformable probabilistic brain atlas based on random vector field transformations. Invited Paper. Med Image Anal 1: 271–294; paper, with video sequences on CD-ROM with Journal Issue, November 1997

Thompson PM, Moussai J, Khan AA, Zohoori S, Goldkorn A, Mega MS, Small GW, Cummings JL, Toga AW (1998) Cortical variability and asymmetry in normal aging and Alzheimer's disease. Cereb Cortex 8:492–509

Thompson PM, Giedd JN, Woods RP, MacDonald D, Evans AC, Toga AW (2000a) Growth patterns in the developing brain detected by using continuum-mechanical tensor maps. Nature 404:190–193

Thompson PM, Mega MS, Narr KL, Sowell ER, Blanton RE, Toga AW (2000b) Brain image analysis and atlas construction. In: Fitzpatrick M (ed) SPIE Handbook on Medical Image Analysis. Society of Photo-Optical Instrumentation Engineers (SPIE) Press

Thompson PM, Mega MS, Toga AW (2000c) Disease-specific brain atlases. In: Toga AW, Mazziotta JC (eds) Brain mapping: the disorders. Academic Press

Thompson PM, Woods RP, Mega MS, Toga AW (2000d) Mathematical/computational challenges in creating population-based brain atlases. Human Brain Mapp 9:81–92

Thompson PM, Cannon TD, Narr KL, van Erp T, Khaledy M, Poutanen V-P, Huttunen M, Lönnqvist J, Standertskjöld-Nordenstam C-G, Kaprio J, Dail R, Zoumalan CI, Toga AW (2001a) Genetic influences on brain structure. Nature Neurosci 4:1253–1258

Thompson PM, de Zubicaray G, Janke AL, Rose SE, Dittmer S, Semple J, Gravano D, Han S, Herman D, Hong MS, Mega MS, Cummings JL, Doddrell DM, Toga AW (2001b) Detecting dynamic (4D) profiles of degenerative rates in Alzheimer's disease patients, using high-resolution tensor mapping and a brain atlas encoding atrophic rates in a population. 7th Annual Meeting of the Organization for Human Brain Mapping, Brighton, England [abstract] 10587

Thompson PM, Mega MS, Vidal C, Rapoport JL, Toga AW (2001c) Detecting disease-specific patterns of brain structure using cortical pattern matching and a population-based probabilistic brain atlas, IEEE Conference on Information Processing in Medical Imaging (IPMI), UC Davis, 2001. In: Insana M, Leahy R (eds) Lecture notes in computer science (LNCS). Springer-Verlag, Heidelberg, 2082:488–501

Thompson PM, Mega MS, Woods RP, Blanton RE, Moussai J, Zoumalan CI, Aron J, Cummings JL, Toga AW (2001d) Early cortical change in Alzheimer's disease detected with a disease-specific population-based brain atlas. Cereb Cortex 11:1–16

Thompson PM, Narr KL, Blanton RE, Toga AW (2001e) Mapping structural alterations of the corpus callosum during brain development and degeneration, In: Iacoboni M, Zaidel E (eds) The corpus callosum. Boston, MIT Press.

Thompson PM, Vidal C, Giedd JN, Gochman P, Blumenthal J, Nicolson R, Toga AW, Rapoport JL (2001f) Mapping adolescent brain change reveals dynamic wave of accelerated gray matter loss in very early-onset schizophrenia. Proc Natl Acad Sci USA 98:11650–11655

Thompson PM, Cannon TD, Toga AW (2002) Mapping genetic influences on human brain structure. Review Paper. Ann Med 34:523–536

Thompson PM, Hayashi KM, de Zubicaray G, Janke AL, Rose SE, Semple J, Doddrell DM, Cannon TD, Toga AW (2002) Detecting dynamic and genetic effects on brain structure using high-dimensional cortical pattern matching. Proc Intl Symp Biomed Imag (ISBI2002), Washington, DC, July 7–10, 2002

Thompson PM, Rapoport JL, Cannon TD, Toga AW (2002c) Imaging the brain as schizophrenia develops: dynamic and genetic brain maps. Invited Paper. Primary Psychiatry 9:40–47

Thompson PM, Hayashi KM, de Zubicaray G, Janke AL, Rose SE, Semple J, Hong MS, Herman D, Gravano D, Dittmer S, Doddrell DM, Toga AW (2003a) Improved detection and mapping of dynamic hippocampal and ventricular change in Alzheimer's disease using 4D parametric mesh skeletonization. 9th Annual Meeting of the Organization for Human Brain Mapping. New York City, NY

Thompson PM, Hayashi KM, de Zubicaray G, Janke AL, Rose SE, Semple J, Herman D, Hong MS, Dittmer SS, Doddrell DM, Toga AW (2003b) Dynamics of gray matter loss in Alzheimer's disease. J Neurosci 23:994–1005

Thompson PM, Rapoport JL, Cannon TD, Toga AW (2003c) Automated analysis of structural MRI data. In: Lawrie AL, Johnstone EC, Weinberger D (eds) Brain imaging in schizophrenia. Oxford, Oxford University Press

Toga AW, Thompson PM (2003a) Mapping brain asymmetry. Nature Rev Neurosci 4:37–48

Toga AW, Thompson PM (2003b) Temporal dynamics of brain anatomy. Ann Rev Biomed Eng, 5:119–145

Uylings HB, de Brabander JM (2002) Neuronal changes in normal human aging and Alzheimer's disease. Brain Cogn 49:268–276

Van Essen DC, Drury HA, Joshi SC, Miller MI (1997) Comparisons between human and macaque using shape-based deformation algorithms applied to cortical flat maps. 3rd Intl Conf Functional Mapping of the Human Brain, Copenhagen, May 19–23, 1997. NeuroImage 5:S41

Vidal CN, Rapoport JL, Gochman P, Giedd JN, Blumenthal J, Gogtay N, Nicolson R, Toga AW, Thompson PM (2003) Mapping lmbic system deficits in adolescents with schizophrenia using novel computational anatomy techniques. 9th Annual Meeting of the Organization for Human Brain Mapping, New York City, NY

Wang D, Chalk JB, Rose SE, de Zubicaray GI, Cowin G, Galloway GJ, Barnes D, Spooner D, Doddrell DM, Semple J (2002) MR image-based measurement of rates of change in volumes of brain structures. Part II: Application to a study of Alzheimer's disease and normal aging. Magn Reson Imag 20:41–48

Weinberger DR, McClure RK (2002) Neurotoxicity, neuroplasticity, and magnetic resonance imaging morphometry: what is happening in the schizophrenic brain? Arch Gen Psychiat 59:553–558

Woods RP (1996) Modeling for intergroup comparisons of imaging data. Neuroimage 4:S84–94

Wright IC, McGuire PK, Poline JB, Travere JM, Murray RM, Frith CD, Frackowiak RSJ, Friston KJ (1995) A voxel-based method for the statistical analysis of gray and white matter density applied to schizophrenia. NeuroImage 2: 244–252

Zeineh MM, Engel SA, Thompson PM, Bookheimer S (2001). Unfolding the human hippocampus with high-resolution structural and functional MRI. Invited Paper. The New Anatomist (Anatomical Record) 265:111–120

Zeineh MM, Engel SA, Thompson PM, Bookheimer SY (2003) Dynamic changes within the human hippocampus during memory consolidation. Science 299:577–580

Zeineh MM, Mazziotta JC, Thompson PM, Engel SA, Bookheimer SY (2003) Hippocampal Flat Maps of Cortical Thickness and Power. 9th Annual Meeting of the Organization for Human Brain Mapping, New York City, NY

Development of Benzothiazole Amyloid-Imaging Agents

William E. Klunk[1], Yanming Wang[1] and Chester A. Mathis[1]

Summary

Alzheimer's disease (AD) is characterized by the widespread deposition of amyloid plaques throughout the neocortex and by neurofibrillary pathology that begins in limbic regions and progresses to cortex. The ability to detect either AD pathology in vivo would have important implications for early diagnosis, deeper understanding of the pathophysiological progression of the disease and assessment of therapies directed specifically at halting these deposits. This chapter describes the work of our laboratory aimed at the development of in vivo positron emission tomography (PET) tracers for use in imaging the pathology of AD. We based these agents on histologic dyes known to bind fibrillar amyloid such as Congo red and thioflavin-T. Assessment of new dye derivatives was guided by criteria borrowed from those used in the development of neuroreceptor PET ligands and further refined during the development of the Congo red class of compounds. Derivatives of the thioflavin-T series are called benzothiazole-aniline, or BTA, compounds. These agents have pharmacokinetic properties similar to successful PET neuroreceptor imaging agents. What's more, the BTA compounds bind to amyloid-beta (Aβ) with high affinity and show very good specificity for amyloid in post-mortem brain preparations. BTA compounds do not appear to bind to neurofibrillary pathology at concentrations commonly attained in PET studies. Analysis of in vitro pharmacologic data and in vivo pharmacokinetic data from animals pointed to a particular hydroxy-BTA compound as the optimal candidate for human PET imaging studies. This compound was termed "Pittsburgh compound B" or "PIB" by our collaborators at the Uppsala University PET Centre, who performed the first human amyloid-imaging studies with PIB in AD patients and controls. That human PET study forms the basis of the chapter by Engler et al. that follows this description of the pre-clinical development of benzothiazole amyloid-imaging agents.

Introduction

The development of biological markers for Alzheimer's disease (AD) has been identified as a priority in the field (Working Group 1998; Growdon 1999). An

---

[1] Departments of Radiology and Psychiatry, University of Pittsburgh, Pittsburgh, Pennsylvania 15213

Hyman et al.
The Living Brain and Alzheimer's
©Springer-Verlag Berlin Heidelberg

ideal biomarker could be used to improve the accuracy of diagnosis in early and confusing presentations of AD. Perhaps more importantly, an ideal biomarker could be used to track the progression of the disease and evaluate the efficacy of therapeutic agents (Working Group 1998; Klunk 1998). Several new therapies targeted at amyloid deposition in AD are in preclinical or early clinical testing (Holtzman et al. 2002; Olson et al. 2001), highlighting the need for new tools to evaluate the efficacy of these new agents.

For example, Figure 1 portrays a hypothetical sequence of events, representative of the "amyloid cascade hypothesis" (Hardy 1992) showing the secretase-mediated cleavage of the amyloid-β (Aβ) precursor protein (APP), oligomer and plaque formation and neurotoxicity. The cause of the neurotoxicity is not certain and may derive from soluble oligomers, fibrillar Aβ or the inflammation associated with Aβ deposits or other sources. Three key therapeutic targets are apparent from this sequence, including 1) modifiers of Aβ metabolism such as secretase inhibitors, 2) Aβ clearing agents, including immunotherapies and aggregation inhibitors and 3) inhibitors of Aβ- or inflammation-induced toxicity. The first target would also include drugs such as non-steroidal anti-inflammatory drugs and statins that may affect the metabolism of APP. In the context of amyloid imaging, the ultimate result of therapeutic agents in the first two categories would be decreased amyloid deposition. Proper evaluation of these "anti-amyloid" therapies will require a method to directly assess brain amyloid burden.

Our approach to the development of amyloid-imaging agents closely follows the approach previously described for the development of neuroreceptor ligands (Eckelman 1989; Eckelman and Gibson 1993; Fig. 2). In this analogy, fibrillar amyloid deposits become the "receptor" or, more properly, the "binding site" target.

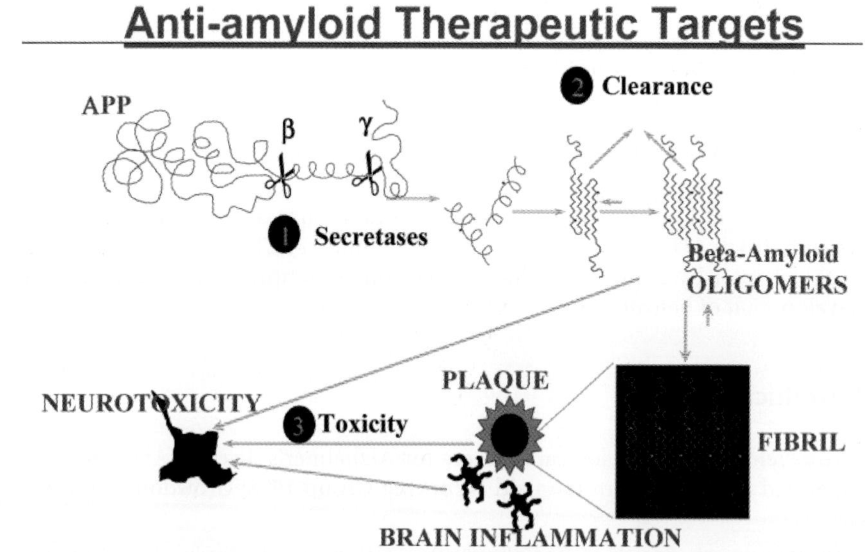

Fig.1. Anti-amyloid therapeutic targets.

Amyloid-Imaging with Positron Emission Tomography (PET): (Bench-to-Bedside)

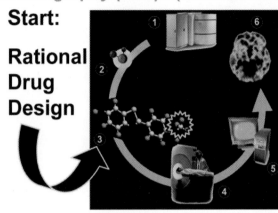

Start:

Rational Drug Design

1. Cyclotron - radionuclide
2. Radiolabeled precursor
3. Radiosynthesis
4. PET Imaging
5. Image Reconstruction
6. Image Analysis

Fig.2. Amyloid-imaging with positron emission tomography (PET). A bench-to-bedside approach.

The choice of the amyloid-imaging "ligand" was the initial, and remained the primary, challenge. This was because of the lack of existing amyloid-binding agents capable of readily entering the brain. In neuroreceptor tracer development, there is often a wealth of tracer candidates to be found among the many non-radioactive compounds developed by pharmaceutical companies in programs of drug development targeted at the receptor of interest. The only corresponding initial information available when our amyloid-imaging program began over a decade ago was the few histologic dyes that were known to bind to amyloid deposits in general (not just Aβ). These dyes included Congo red, thioflavin-S and thioflavin-T (Klunk et al. 2001).

The goal for amyloid imaging can be exemplified by previously successful neuroreceptor positron emission tomography (PET) imaging studies (Fig. 3). The time-activity curves on the left of Figure 3 demonstrate how a good neuroimaging agent [in this case [carbonyl-^{11}C]WAY 100635, a serotonin 5-HT$_{1A}$ receptor ligand] enters all areas of the brain rapidly and clears rapidly from brain areas having few receptor sites [e.g., cerebellum (CER)], but is retained for longer periods in brain areas rich in binding sites [e.g., medial temporal cortex (MTC)]. This behavior results in specific binding of the receptors of interest with good signal-to-noise.

Contained in the behavior of this radiotracer imaging agent are the following criteria, which we have borrowed from neuroreceptor development and modified slightly for the development of amyloid-imaging agents:

1. The tracer must bind to its target (i.e., amyloid) with high affinity (Kd or Ki < 10 nM). This allows the compound to be retained in brain areas rich in tar-

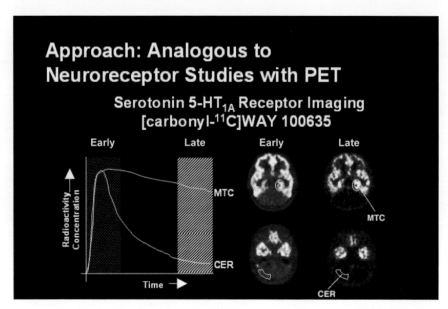

Fig.3. Our approach toward amyloid-imaging agents is very similar to the approach toward development of neuroreceptor ligands. Shown here are time-activity curves and PET images from a very good neuroreceptor imaging agent. Note good brain entry into both cerebellum (CER, which does not contain 5-HT$_{1A}$ binding sites) and medial temporal cortex (MTC, which is rich in 5-HT$_{1A}$ binding sites) at early time points. This is followed by rapid clearance of the tracer from CER but retention in MTC, providing a measure of the relative number of binding sites in each tissue.

get (e.g., amyloid deposits) while free and non-specifically bound tracers are washed away from brain areas with few binding sites.

2. Rapid attainment of high concentrations in all areas of the brain. This must occur rapidly because of the short half-lives of PET radiotracers (20 min in the case of carbon-11). It is important to define a quantifiable goal for brain entry, rather than just state that a compound "enters the brain." This goal is necessitated by the sensitivity limit of the detection technique (in this case PET) and can be defined from the behavior of previously successful neuroimaging agents. It appears necessary for ~0.5% of the total injected dose (ID) to enter the whole brain in a typical 200-g rat. Normalizing this value derived from rat studies by the brain-to-body weight ratio yields what we have termed the percent injected dose index (or %IDI). In these units, which apply to any species including humans, a brain level of approximately 100 %IDI [equivalent to 0.10 (%ID)/g/kg body weight] of a given tracer must initially enter the brain to provide adequate detection by PET.

3. Clearance of free and non-specifically bound tracer must occur quickly. How quickly depends on the half-life of the tracer used, but the clearance half-time of the tracer from non-target areas of the brain should typically be no greater than 30 min for PET ligands (with periods below 10 min even better for carbon-

11 compounds). Inherent in this property is the criterion that the non-specific binding of radiotracer be low. A high level of non-specific binding in vivo is a common cause of radiotracer failure. Therefore, the specificity of our lead compounds will be discussed in more detail below.

Summary of Congo Red Derivatives

As stated above, our group has worked for many years on the development of Congo red derivatives, incrementally approaching our goals for affinity and brain entry and clearance. Figure 4 summarizes the four generations of Congo red derivatives developed. The first generation prototype is Congo red itself. These compounds are characterized by azo groups (N=N) and highly charged sulfonic acids. The sulfonic acid prevents Congo red from entering the brain in amounts sufficient for detection by PET (%IDI < 10) (Tubis et al. 1960). The second generation of Congo red compounds is typified by Chrysamine-G. These compounds also have the azo linkage, but replace the naphthalene sulfonic acid moieties with more lipophilic salicylic acid groups. Radiolabeled Chrysamine-G derivatives have not been found to enter the brain in amounts sufficient for PET imaging

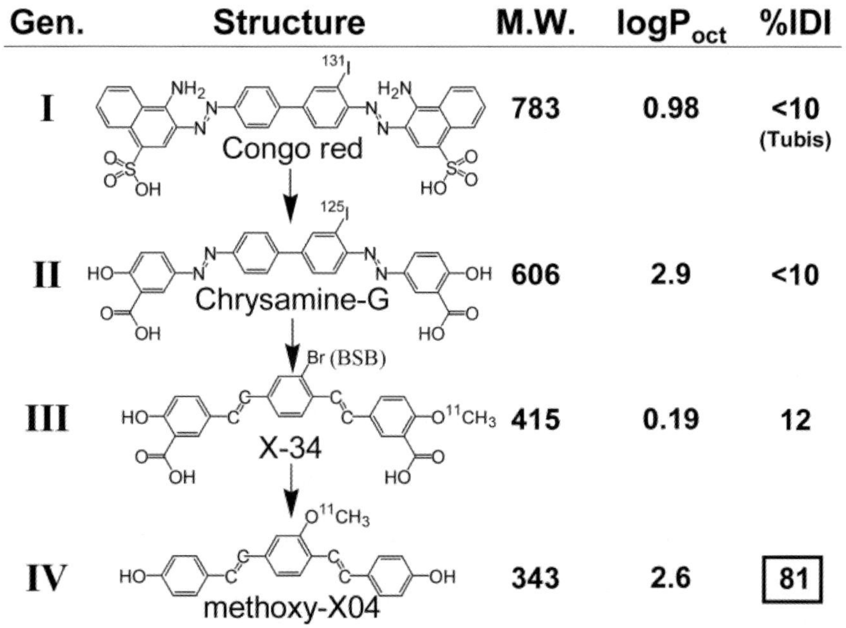

Gen.	Structure	M.W.	logP$_{oct}$	%IDI
I	Congo red	783	0.98	<10 (Tubis)
II	Chrysamine-G	606	2.9	<10
III	X-34	415	0.19	12
IV	methoxy-X04	343	2.6	81

Fig.4. Structures of examples from four "generations" of Congo red derivatives. Also shown are the molecular weights (M.W.), a measure of lipophilicity, the log$_{10}$ of the octanol-water partition coefficient (logP$_{oct}$), and the degree of brain entry at 2 min post i.v. injection in terms of %IDI (see text).

(Mathis et al. 1997; Zhen et al. 1999; Dezutter et al. 1999). The third generation of Congo red derivatives is characterized by replacement of the azo linker with an alkene group (C=C). The salicylic acids are retained. Despite a decrease in molecular weight (a factor known to aid brain entry; Levin 1980), members of this group achieved only slightly better brain entry than second-generation compounds. Suspecting that the carboxylic acids were the source of the poor brain entry, we synthesized and tested a fourth generation of compounds with only the very weakly acidic phenols. Several compounds in this group showed significantly improved brain entry (Klunk et al. 2002; Wang et al. 2002). Multiphoton microscopy studies performed in living transgenic mice using methoxy-X04 (Fig. 4) showed in vivo labeling of individual amyloid plaques by this fluorescent compound. Methoxy-X04 approached our brain entry criteria of 100 %IDI, achieving 81 %IDI, but the clearance half-time of this compound was just over 30 min. The compound was judged to be marginally acceptable as an in vivo amyloid-imaging agent for human PET studies. It does, however, appear well suited for multiphoton microscopic imaging studies in transgenic mice (Klunk et al. 2002).

Thioflavin-T Derivatives: BTA Compounds

In considering possible pharmacophores outside of the Congo red class of compounds upon which to base the development of amyloid-imaging PET agents, we began a program built around thioflavin-T derivatives (Klunk et al. 2001). Building on the insights learned through the four generations of Congo red derivatives, our initial chemical modifications were targeted at removing the positive charge inherent in the thioflavin-T parent compound (Fig. 5).

The basic backbone of these thioflavin-T derivatives is composed of a benzothiazole group connected to an aniline group. A shorthand nomenclature was developed, calling the class "BTA" for benzothiazole-aniline. The position and type of substituent on the benzothiazole portion are noted before "BTA" and the number of methyl groups on the aniline nitrogen is noted after "BTA." Thus, 6-Me-BTA-2 refers to a BTA compound with a six-position methyl group and two methyl substituents on the aniline nitrogen. As a group, these BTA compounds entered the brain very well, achieving 2-min brain levels between 200 and 500 %IDI. They bound to amyloid fibrils with good affinity (many with a Ki < 10 nM). A structure-activity survey of BTA compounds showed that the free and nonspecifically bound components of many compounds cleared very well (Mathis et al. 2003). Thus several BTA compounds met affinity and brain entry/clearance criteria predicted to be necessary for good amyloid-imaging agents.

A major factor still to be determined was the specificity of this class of compounds for amyloid. For evaluation of this question, we chose the prototypical BTA compound, 2-(4'-methylaminophenyl)benzothiazole (BTA-1; Klunk et al. 2003). As a first, crude measure of specificity, the ability of BTA-1 to specifically stain amyloid deposits in post-mortem tissue was determined. This is an approximate method because the concentrations used (1 µM) are 1000-fold greater than those utilized in PET studies. At 1 µM, BTA-1 stained amyloid plaques, cerebrovascular amyloid and neurofibrillary tangles. However, when binding was studied

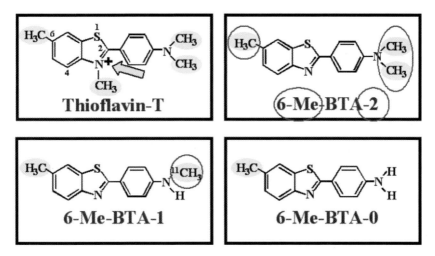

Fig.5. Structures of the first thioflavin-T derivatives studied. The arrow points to the benzothiazolium nitrogen with the positive charge in thioflavin-T. The gray ovals highlight the various methyl substituents. Circles highlight the details used in our shorthand nomenclature (see text), which results in the names of the compounds noted below each structure.

in homogenates of AD brain tissue at [^{3}H]BTA-1 concentrations more similar to those attained in in vivo PET studies (1 nM), clear evidence of binding to Aβ deposits in neocortex was present, but there was no significant binding to tissues that contained neurofibrillary tangles but no plaques [e.g., transentorhinal cortex from a Braak stage II control brain (Braak and Braak 1991; Klunk et al. 2003). This finding suggests that in vivo binding of BTA compounds would mainly be a reflection of plaque and cerebrovascular amyloid deposits.

Further study of homogenates of frontal cortex from AD and control brain showed that the binding of [^{3}H]BTA-1, and several other BTA derivatives, to synthetic Aβ fibrils was over 90% specific (i.e., displaceable by excess non-radioactive compound; Klunk et al., 2003). Consistent with this finding, the absolute amount of BTA-1 bound to brain homogenates from AD brain (in terms of pmol BTA-1 bound per mg tissue) was 10-fold greater than the amount bound to brain homogenates from age-matched, cognitively normal controls or non-AD dementia controls. More detailed study revealed that high-affinity BTA-1 binding sites were found only in the gray matter of AD brain, not in underlying white matter. Interestingly, for a wide variety of BTA compounds spanning a 1000-fold range of binding affinity to synthetic Aβ, the binding affinity determined in AD brain homogenates closely matched that determined in synthetic Aβ preparations (r=0.88; Klunk et al. 2003). Taken together, these data represent strong support for the hypothesis that the binding of BTA derivatives to AD brain largely reflects the Aβ content of that brain tissue. This hypothesis was further supported by multiphoton microscopic studies in transgenic mouse models of AD. With the 1-micron resolution of multiphoton microscopy, individual plaques and cerebrovascular amyloid labeled by BTA-1 could be easily detected (Mathis et al. 2002).

At this point, it seemed like the BTA class of compounds contained several agents that met our criteria for an acceptable amyloid-imaging agent. The task then became choosing the lead compound that would optimize the chances of success in human PET neuroimaging studies. Several compounds were considered, but two compounds appeared to be the most promising. These were BTA-1 and its hydroxylated derivative, 2-(4'-methylaminophenyl)-6-hydroxybenzothiazole (6-OH-BTA-1). Both of these compounds (and radiolabeling precursors) were sent to the Uppsala University PET Centre (UUPC) for consideration of human studies and were given the UUPC codes PIA (BTA-1) and PIB (6-OH-BTA-1) for "Pittsburgh A" and "Pittsburgh B." Prior to the final choice, a decision was made to carefully compare the pharmacokinetic properties of these compounds in primate cerebellum in comparison to other known useful PET neuroreceptor imaging agents (including [carbonyl-^{11}C]WAY 100635 and [^{18}F]altanserin; Mathis et al. 2003).

The cerebellum was chosen because of the known scarcity of fibrillar amyloid deposits in this area, along with the absence of serotonin- or dopamine-binding sites. This means that this comparison is limited to prediction of the pharmacokinetics of free and non-specifically bound radiotracer and overlooks the behavior of specifically bound tracer since there are no Aβ binding sites in primate cerebellum. Figure 6 shows that three of the most useful PET neuroreceptor imaging agents in common use at the University of Pittsburgh Medical Center PET Facility ([^{18}F]altanserin, [^{11}C]raclopride and [carbonyl-^{11}C]WAY 100635) define a target range for the pharmacokinetic behavior of PET neuroreceptor radiotracers. When BTA-1 and the 6-hydroxy derivative are compared in this way, [^{11}C]6-OH-BTA-1 falls into the target range both by uptake and clearance criteria whereas BTA-1

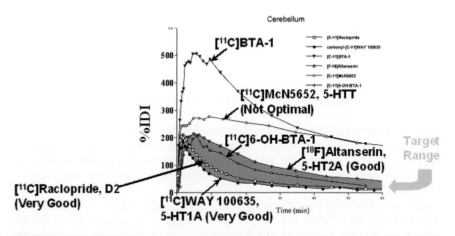

Fig.6. Baboon cerebellar entry and clearance of radiotracers commonly used in the University of Pittsburgh Medical Center PET Facility. Also shown for comparison are the time-activity curves of [^{11}C]BTA-1 and [^{11}C]6-OH-BTA-1. Note the gray target range defined by the currently successful compounds. Only [^{11}C]6-OH-BTA-1 falls into this range.

does not. The failure of BTA-1 to fit this target range is due to both increased uptake (not a negative finding in itself) and decreased clearance rate.

With the choice of the lead amyloid-imaging agent made, the Uppsala University group proceeded with a microdosing toxicology study (Bergström et al. 2003; Lappin and Garner 2003). This study showed no significant toxic effects of the 6-hydroxy derivative, PIB. Human PIB imaging studies were initiated in February 2002 and form the subject for the chapter in this text by Dr. Engler and his colleagues at the Uppsala University PET Centre. Similar studies, producing very similar findings, began in February 2003 at the University of Pittsburgh PET Facility.

In summary, benzothiazole amyloid-imaging agents were developed by iterative modification of the parent compound, thioflavin-T. Choices regarding the most useful derivatives were guided by criteria borrowed largely from neuroreceptor ligand development and refined during development of the Congo red class of amyloid-imaging agents. The development of the BTA class of compounds proceeded fairly quickly (taking just over two years from outset to first human study) but was catalyzed to a great extent by the structure-activity experience gained during the previous decade of work on four generations of Congo red derivatives. The lessons learned and criteria refined during the development of the Congo red and BTA classes of amyloid-imaging agents should be fairly general and apply to the development of other amyloid-imaging agents intended for detection by techniques other than PET (such a SPECT and perhaps MRI). These criteria are currently being applied to the development of fluorine-18-labeled BTA derivatives, which have the advantage of a 110-min radioactive half-life. However, the 6-hydroxy BTA derivative, commonly termed PIB, appears to be a useful amyloid-imaging agent that should be able to contribute to better understanding of the pathophysiology of AD, lead to improved early diagnosis and aid in the development of anti-amyloid therapeutic drugs. In addition, the 20-min half-life of the carbon-11 label of PIB allows multiple, sequential PET studies in a single scanning session, such as PIB followed by [^{18}F]fluorodeoxyglucose.

References

Bergström M, Grahnén A, Långström B (2003) PET-microdosing, a new concept with application in early clinical drug development. Eur J Clin Pharmacol 59:357–366
Braak H, Braak E (1991) Neuropathological staging of Alzheimer-related changes. Acta Neuropathol 82:239–259
Dezutter NA, Dom RJ, de Groot TJ, Bormans GM, Verbruggen AM (1999) 99mTc-MAMA-chrysamine G, a probe for beta-amyloid protein of Alzheimer's disease. Eur J Nucl Med 26:1392–1399
Eckelman WC (1989) The use of in vitro models to predict the distribution of receptor binding radiotracers in vivo. Intl J Rad Appl Instrument Part B Nucl Med Biol 16:233–245
EckelmanWC, Gibson RE (1993) The design of site-directed radiopharmaceuticals for use in drug discovery. In: Burns HD, Gibson RE, Dannals RF, Siegl PK, Burns DH (eds) Nuclear imaging in drug discovery, development and approval. Birkhäuser, Boston, pp. 113–134
Growdon JH (1999) Biomarkers of Alzheimer disease. Arch Neurol 56:281-283
Hardy J (1992) An 'anatomical cascade hypothesis' for Alzheimer's disease. Trends Neurosci 15:200–201

Holtzman DM, Bales KR, Paul SM, DeMattos RB (2002) Abeta immunization and Anti-Abeta antibodies: potential therapies for the prevention and treatment of Alzheimer's disease. Adv Drug Deliv Rev 54:1603–1613

Klunk WE (1998) Biological markers of Alzheimer's disease. Neurobiol Aging 19:145–147

Klunk WE, Wang Y, Huang G-F, Debnath ML, Holt DP, Mathis CA (2001) Uncharged thioflavin-T derivatives bind to amyloid-beta protein with high affinity and readily enter the brain. Life Sci 69:1471–1484

Klunk WE, Bacskai BJ, Mathis CA, Kajdasz ST, Mclellan ME, Frosch MP, Debnath ML, Holt DP, Wang Y, Hyman BT (2002) Imaging Abeta plaques in living transgenic mice with multi-photon microscopy and methoxy-X04, a systemically administered Congo red derivative. J Neuropathol Exp Neurol 61:797–805

Klunk WE, Wang Y, Huang G-F, Debnath ML, Holt DP, Shao L, Hamilton RL, Ikonomovic MD, DeKosky ST, Mathis CA (2003) The binding of 2-(4'-Methylaminophenyl)Benzothiazole to post-mortem brain homogenates is dominated by the amyloid component. J Neurosci 23:2086–2092

Lappin G, Garner RC (2003) Big physics, small doses: the use of AMS and PET in human micro-dosing of development drugs. Nature Rev 2:233–240

Levin VA (1980) Relationship of octanol/water partition coefficient and molecular weight to rat brain capillary permeability. J Med Chem 23:682–684

Mathis CA, Mahmood K, Debnath ML, Klunk WE (1997) Synthesis of a lipophilic radioiodina-ted ligand with high affinity to amyloid protein in Alzheimer's disease brain tissue. J Label Compds Radiopharmacol 40:94–95

Mathis CA, Bacskai BJ, Kajdasz ST, Mclellan ME, Frosch MP, Hyman BT, Holt DP, Wang Y, Huang G-F, Debnath ML, Klunk WE (2002) A lipophilic thioflavin-T derivative for positron emission tomography (PET) imaging of amyloid in brain. Bioorg Med Chem Lett 12:295–298

Mathis CA, Wang Y, Holt DP, Huang G-F, Debnath ML, Klunk WE (2003) Synthesis and eva-luation of ^{11}C-labeled 6-substituted 2-aryl benzothiazoles as amyloid imaging agents. J Med Chem 46:2740–2754

Olson RE, Copeland RA, Seiffert D (2001) Progress towards testing the amyloid hypothesis: in-hibitors of APP processing. Curr Opin Drug Disc Dev 4:390–401

Tubis M, Blahd WH, Nordyke RA (1960) The preparation and use of radioiodinated Congo red in detecting amyloidosis. J Am Pharmaceut Assoc 49:422–425

Wang Y, Mathis CA , Huang,G-F, Holt DP, Debnath ML, Klunk WE (2002) Synthesis and ^{11}C-la-belling of (E,E)-1-(3',4'-dihydroxystyryl)-4-(3'-methoxy-4'-hydroxystyryl) benzene for PET imaging of amyloid deposits. J Label Compd Radiopharmacol 45:647–664

Working Group (1998) Consensus report of the Working Group on: "Molecular and Biochemi-cal Markers of Alzheimer's Disease". The Ronald and Nancy Reagan Research Institute of the Alzheimer's Association and the National Institute on Aging Working Group. Neurobiol Aging 19:109–116

Zhen W, Han H, Anguiano M, Lemere CA, Cho CG, Lansbury PT (1999) Synthesis and amyloid binding properties of rhenium complexes: preliminary progress toward a reagent for SPECT imaging of Alzheimer's disease brain. J Med Chem 42:2805–2815

First PET Study with a Benzothiazol Amyloid-imaging Agent (PIB) in Alzheimer's Disease Patients and Healthy Volunteers

Henry Engler[1], William Klunk[3], Agneta Nordberg[2], Gunnar Blomqvist[1], Daniel Holt[3], Yanming Wang[3], Mats Bergström[1], Guo-feng Huang[3], Sergio Estrada[1], Manik Debnath[3], Julien Barletta[4], Johan Sandell[1] Anders Wall[1],Gunnar Antoni[1], Chester Mathis[3], Bengt Långström[1,4]

Summary

Amyloid plaques are a hallmark of Alzheimer's disease (AD) and have become a therapeutic target, creating a need to quantify plaque deposition in vivo. Recently, benzothiazole-aniline derivatives that bind amyloid-beta protein with high affinity and cross the blood–brain barrier have been developed. These have been characterized by pre-clinical pharmacology and toxicology, resulting in the choice of [N-methyl-^{11}C]2-[4'-(methylamino)-phenyl]6-hydroxybenzothiazole, [(6-OH-BTA-1) = PIB, according to the Uppsala University code] for the first human study with positron emission tomography (PET).

Nine patients with the clinical diagnosis of AD and five healthy volunteers were examined using a dual tracer protocol consisting of ^{18}F-labelled deoxyglucose (FDG) and PIB. The objective of the study was to determine the distribution of PIB in the brains of AD patients and healthy volunteers and compare this distribution to the cerebral metabolic rate in both groups.

In AD patients, PIB was retained in frontal and temporoparietal association cortices. Low retention was observed in the sensorimotor cortex, the visual cortex, the thalami, the brainstem, the putamen and the cerebellum. In the healthy volunteers, the uptake was very low in every cortical area.

Some correlation between the localization of PIB and the areas of hypometabolism was found in the AD patients. The distribution of PIB in the patients is consistent with the known topology of amyloid plaque deposition in AD brain.

This tracer seems to be a promising human amyloid-imaging agent, which appears to have good specificity for amyloid deposits in vivo. This new approach might have important diagnostic uses and might serve as a surrogate marker for evaluating the efficacy of anti-amyloid therapeutics that are already used in clinical trials.

[1] Uppsala Univ. PET Centre/Uppsala IMANET AB, Uppsala, Sweden
[2] Geriatric Department, Karolinska Institute, Huddinge University Hospital, Srockholm, Sweden,
[3] Univ. of Pittsburgh, Pittsburgh, Pennsylvania, USA
[4] Department of Organic Chemistry, Uppsala University, Uppsala, Sweden

Hyman et al.
The Living Brain and Alzheimer's
©Springer-Verlag Berlin Heidelberg

Introduction

Alzheimer's disease (AD) is the most common form of dementia, characterized by an insidious onset and a gradual loss of memory and other cognitive abilities. Accompanying the aging of the world population, there is a massive increase in the number of people affected by AD. Despite a rapid increase in our knowledge of the underlying pathophysiological processes of the disease, there is still no cure. AD is characterized by two types of protein aggregates, the neurofibrillary tangles and amyloid plaques, which are distributed in regions of the brain that are involved in learning and memory (Braak and Braak1991). The neurofibrillary tangles consist of twisted filaments containing hyperphoshorylated tau whereas the amyloid plaques contain ß-amyloid (Aß) peptide fibrils. The cloning of a gene encoding the ß-amyloid precursor protein (APP) and its localization to chromosome 21 created the Aß cascade hypothesis as a primary event in AD pathology (Hardy and Allsop 1991).

So far a definitive diagnosis based on a histopathological demonstration of amyloid plaques and neurofibrillary tangles can only be made at autopsy. An in vivo amyloid imaging technology could thus fill the need for an accurate diagnostic tool in very early and perhaps presymptomatic stages of AD. This technology would also allow early initiation of drug therapy. It is quite obvious that early detection of the disease will be a prerequisite for the emerging new drug treatment strategies in AD.

Many efforts have been made to develop amyloid-imaging agents for PET, SPECT and MRI (Klunk et al. 1999; Agdeppa et al. 2001; Dezutter et al. 2001; Friedland et al. 1997; Shoghi-Jadid et al. 2002), etc. Many early agents were hampered by poor brain entry. The discovery of the benzothiazole class of amyloid-binding compounds led to agents that crossed the blood-brain barrier very well (Klunk et al. 2001).The basic properties of the simplest benzothiazole amyloid binding agent, [N-methyl-C-11]2-(4'-methylaminophenyl)-benzothiazole, have been described in detail (Mathis, et al. 2003). These compounds could bind to amyloid with low nanomolar affinity, enter brain in amounts sufficient for PET imaging, bind specifically to amyloid deposits in the brain, and clear rapidly from normal tissue. A structure-activity study of a series of benzothiazoles suggested that a hydroxylated derivative, [N-methyl-C-11]2-(4'-methylaminophenol)-6-hydroxy-benzothiazole, had better brain clearance properties for in vivo PET application (Mathis et al. 2003). Therefore, this hydroxybenzothiazole was chosen as the lead compound for the first human trial of benzothiazole amyloid-imaging agents. For simplicity, the compound was given the Uppsala University PET Centre code of "Pittsburgh Compound-B" or simply PIB.

This study describes the preliminary results from PET imaging of nine mild AD patients and five healthy controls. A robust difference between the PIB labelling patterns in cortical brain regions was observed in the AD patients compared to healthy controls.

Materials and methods Radio tracers

^{18}F-FDG was produced according to the standard GMP at the Uppsala

Synthesis of PIB

[^{11}C]carbon dioxide was produced by the ^{14}N(p,_)^{11}C reaction using the MC17 cyclotron (Scanditronix, Uppsala, Sweden) at the Uppsala University PET Centre. PIB was prepared from the methoxy-protected precursor 4-(6-methoxymethoxy-benzothiazol-2-yl)-phenylamine in two radiochemical steps (scheme 1). The precursor (0.5 mg, 1.7 µmol) and NaH (0.4 mg, 16 µmol) were dissolved in DMF (200 µL) in a 0.9 mL mini-vial. The mini-vial was sealed and the mixture was shaken for 2 min, after which it turned yellow. [^{11}C]Methyl iodide was trapped at ambient temperature and the reaction was heated at around 100°C for 3 min. Deprotection was achieved by adding HCl/MeOH (1/2, 200 µL) and subsequent heating for an additional 5 min at 120°C. The mixture was diluted with 500 µL HPLC mobile phase prior to injection onto the semi-preparative HPLC column [Column: Ultrasphere ODS, C18, 5mm, 250 mm'10 mm i.d., eluted with 50 mM aqueous ammonium formate at pH 3.5 (solvent A) and acetonitrile–water (50:7, v/v) (solvent B), a linear gradient from 40% to 65% B over 20 min, flow rate 6 ml/min]. The radioactive fraction containing PIB was collected (retention time 11.5 min), and after evaporation of the mobile phase the residue was re-dissolved in 4 mL of a sterile mixture consisting of saline (2 mL, NaCl 9 mg/ml), propyleneglycol (2 mL), ethanol (0.7 mL) and HCl (0.3 mL, 0.3 mM). The residue was subsequently filtered (Dynagard ME, 0.22 µm) into a sterile injection flask yielding a solution that was sterile and free from pyrogens. Addition of 5 mL sterile phosphate-buffered saline to the solution adjusted the pH to between 6 and 7. The incorporation of [^{11}C]methyl iodide to [^{11}C]PIB was in the range of 10-15% and the specific radioactivity was on average 25 GBq/µmol (range 6-74) at the end of synthesis.

Quality management

Routine quality control of the injection solution consisted of a measurement of the pH and by HPLC analysis of the radiochemical and chemical purity [20 µL injected, Column: Ultrasphere ODS, 250 mm'4.6 mm i.d. eluted with 50 mM aqueous ammonium formate at pH 3.5 (solvent A) and acetonitrile–water, (50:7, v/v) (solvent B), at 40% B, for 2 min, and then a linear gradient from 40% to 70% over 10 min, flow rate 2 ml/min. UV-detection at 254 nm]. The retention time of PIB was 5.0 min and the radiochemical purity was generally better than 95%.

In addition, the following analyses were performed on selected batches: sterility and endotoxin tests, radiochemical and chemical stability tests, including column recovery determination, and verification of the identity of the radiolabelled compound with LC-MS.

The human use of PIB was associated with a toxicity assessment using our PET-microdosing concept (Bergström et al. 2003). This implies that a PET tracer, which is given with the non-radioactive counterpart in doses of a few micrograms, need not undergo the same extensive toxicity assessment as drugs in clinical trials, which typically are given in mg quantities.

AD Patients

Nine patients (three females and six males) ranging in age from 51 to 80 years of age (mean age 63 ± 11, Mv ± SD) were recruited to the study at the Geriatric Medicine Department, Huddinge University Hospital, Karolinska Institute, Stockholm. The patients had been diagnosed with probable AD according to the criteria of NINCDS-ADRDA (McKhann et al. 1984). The diagnosis was made after a comprehensive clinical examination, including a medical history with a close informant, neurological and psychiatric examinations, routine blood analysis, ECG, MRI /CT scans, SPECT scans, EEG, CSF sampling with tau analysis, Apolipoprotein E (APOE) genotyping and a comprehensive neuropsychological examination. The degrees of dementia, as evaluated by the Mini-Mental-State-Examination (MMSE) scores, varied from mild to very mild, ranging from 18-28 (mean ± SD,

Table 1. Demographic data for AD patients and control subjects. Mean values ± SD

	AD	Controls
N (female/male)	9 (3/6)	5 (4/1)
Age (Mv ± SD) (years)	62.3 ± 9.3	69.9 ± 6.5
Range	51–80	21–67
ApoE e4/e3	4/5	
MMSE (/30)	23.3 ± 3.7	30
Range	18–28	
Tau (pg/ml)	597 21 ± 130	
Range	329–1180	
Aß 1-42 (pg/ml)	394 ± 130	
Range	329–1180	
Duration of disease (years)	4.3 ± 2.0	
Range	1–7	
Time since diagnostis	0.2–6	

23.3 ± 3.7). The duration of the disease varied from 1-7 years (mean ±SD, 4.3 ± 2.0 years), and the length of time since diagnosis was 0.2-6 years (mean ± SD, 2.5 ±2.2 years). Five of the patients (one female, three males) had been on cholinesterase inhibitor treatment (rivastigmine) for three to four years (mean ± SD, 3.8 ± 0.4 years), whereas four patients who had been diagnosed recently were not on cholinesterase inhibitor treatment. CSF tau value was 597 ± 313 pg/ml (329-1180) and beta amyloid (Aß 1-42) was 394 ± 130 pg/ml (143- 589) and thus within reference interval for AD patients (Table 1). All patients and their next of kin gave informed consent to participate in the study. The study was approved by the Ethics Committee of Uppsala University and Karolinska Insitutet, Stockholm, and the Isotope Committee, Uppsala University Hospital, Uppsala, Sweden.

Healthy control subjects

Five subjects, two aged 59 and 67 (one male and one female) and three females 21 years of age, volunteered as normal controls for regional brain glucose metabolic rate, $rCMR_{glu}$ and determination of their PIB slope values. None of the healthy volunteers had a history of a medical or neurological disease or substance abuse. The two older control subjects were spouses of two of the patients. They underwent neuropsychological testing with normal performances. The younger controls were psychology students with no known cognitive impairments. They were studied under a separate Human Ethics Committee Protocol, which included an arterial line for the purposes of validating the use of the cerebellum as a reference region. These subjects were also chosen because of the very small probability of inadvertently including an amyloid-positive, pre-clinical case of AD in this young age group.

Positron emission tomography

Procedure

Patients and healthy volunteers were examined after at least a six-hour fasting period before PET. Electrocardiography, pulse and blood pressure were measured throughout the examination with PIB.

PET Scanning

PET was performed in two Siemens ECAT HR+ cameras with an axial field of view of 155 mm, providing 63 contiguous 2.46 mm slices with a 5.6 mm transaxial and a 5.4 mm axial resolution. The orbito-meatal line was used to center the head of the subjects.

The patients and healthy volunteers were given iv injections of approximately 300 MBq of PIB. PET measured the time-dependent uptake of radioactivity in the brain according to a predetermined set of measurements (Frames, 2 x 60 s, 3 x 120 s, 4 x 180 s, 4 x 300 s and 2 x 600 s) for one hour.

Arterialized blood samples were obtained from nine patients and two age-matched controls. Arterial blood samples from the radial artery could only be obtained in two of the three young healthy volunteers. Subjects were given 200-300 MBq of ^{18}F-FDG iv and PET measured the radioactivity in the brain for 5 x 60, 5 x 180, 5 x 300 and 1 x 600 seconds frames for 55 minutes. The plasma glucose concentration was measured three times, once before and two times after the ^{18}F-FDG injections.

The scans were corrected for scatter and attenuation using a transmission scan for 10 minutes and were reconstructed using a backprojection and a Hanning filter 4. A computerized re-orientation procedure was used to align consecutive PET studies for accurate intra- and interindividual comparisons (Andersson and Thurfjell 1997).

Regions of interest

All PET investigations were analyzed using identical standardized regions of interest (ROIs) in the brain (Engler,et al. 2003)

Kinetic analysis of the data

A modification of the original Patlak method for reference tissue with reference tissue (Patlak, and Blasberg 1985) was used for the quantitative analysis of the PIB data (Blomqvist et al. 2002). With PIB there is irreversible accumulation of tracer in all regions, precluding the use of the total uptake, $C_S^{ref}(t)$, in the reference region. Instead the concentration of free tracer in the reference tissue, $C_F^{ref}(t)$, is used as reference. Assuming that the model with one reversible and one irreversible compartment (three rate constants) is valid, $C_F^{ref}(t)$ is estimated from the measured $C_S^{ref}(t)$, and knowledge of the rate constant l_3 for the irreversible binding in the reference tissue, a plot of $C_S^{tar}(t)/C_S^{ref}(t)$ versus $\int_0^t C_S^{ref}(x)dx/C_S^{ref}(t)$, gives asymptotically a straight line with slope

$$(k_2 + Rl_3)k_3/(k_2+k_3) \tag{1}$$

Here $C_S^{tar}(t)$ is the time-activity in the target region, k_2 is the rate constant for efflux from the brain back to blood, and k_3 is the rate constant for binding in the target region. R is the ratio between the influx rate constants in the target and reference regions. If $k_2 >> k_3$ and $k_2 >> Rl_3$, the slope is close to k_3. It is assumed that k_3 for PIB is proportional to the concentration of $A\beta$.

The accumulation rate constant l3 was obtained from the two experiments, where the time-activity in arterial plasma corrected for labelled metabolites was determined. The cerebellum was chosen as reference region, because it is expected that the accumulation of PIB in this region does not differ substantially between the healthy control and AD groups.

Parametric maps of the slope obtained from the reference-Patlak analysis were constructed, In this case the original and not the corrected reference tissue method was applied. The effect of not correcting for the irreversible accumulation in the reference tissue is most prominent in regions with low accumulation.

Metabolite Analysis

Whole blood samples were centrifuged and equal amounts of acetonitrile were added to the plasma fraction to precipitate the proteins. The protein-free fraction was analyzed by HPLC. Separation of metabolites and tracer was performed on a Genesis C18 column with a mobile phase consisting of acetonitrile-50 mM ammoniumformate, pH 3.5 (55:45, v/v). The metabolite and tracer fractions were collected and the radioactivity was measured in a well-type scintillation counter.

FDG

Parametric maps of glucose metabolic rate (CMR_{glc}) were generated by the Patlak-technique using the time course of the tracer in arterialized venous plasma as input function (Gjedde 1981; Patlak and Blasberg 1983). In an attempt to reduce intersubject variability, the values of glucose metabolic rate were normalized to the metabolic rate in the sensorimotorcortex to calculate a glucose metabolic index (Raichle et al. 1983). Taking advantage of the 20-min half-life of carbon-11, FDG scans could be performed 120 minutes after the injection of PIB.

Results

The uptake to brain of PIB was studied in five healthy subjects and nine AD patients. The healthy controls showed rapid uptake and clearance of PIB in all cortical and subcortical areas containing gray matter and cerebellum (Fig. 1). In contrast, the white matter showed a relatively lower uptake and slower clearance. In spite of small quantitative differences, the two older healthy controls showed a pattern similar to that found in the young controls. Both groups were therefore combined as the healthy control group (HC) for comparison to the AD group.

The AD patients showed a marked retention of PIB in areas of the brain known to contain large amounts of amyloid deposits, such as association cortex including temporal, parietal and frontal cortices (Arnold et al.1991). Retention was low in areas known to be relatively unaffected by amyloid deposition, such as brain stem, cerebellum, the thalami and sensorimotor cortex in the AD patients (Fig. 1).

The white matter and the cerebellum showed similar clearance of the compound in AD patients and healthy volunteers. Clearance in amyloid-containing areas of AD patients was significantly slower than that seen in HC (Fig. 1).

Figure 2 shows maps of slope obtained with the reference-Patlak method for a) one HC subject and b) one AD patient. The pattern of accumulation was almost

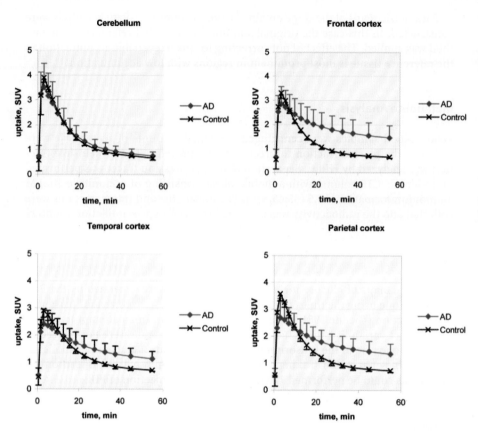

Fig. 1. Uptake of PIB in four brain regions in healthy control (HC) subjects (young, old) and AD patients. HC, n=5,;AD, n=9.

inverse in the AD patient compared to the HC subject, with PIB accumulation in the AD patient being most prominent in cortical areas and lower in white matter areas, whereas HC images showed almost no imaging in cortical areas, leaving the subcortical white matter regions highest in relative terms. It is important to emphasize that the accumulation rate of tracer in white matter was essentially the same in AD and HC subjects.

In the two experiments with arterial sampling, the original Gjedde-Patlak method using plasma input function was applied. The plots show that the uptake is compatible with irreversible accumulation of the tracer in all areas during the measured time (60 min). A very low accumulation was observed in the reference region, the cerebellum. Applying the kinetic model with one reversible and one irreversible compartment to these two experiments, good fits to the data were obtained in all regions. In the cerebellum the rate-constant, k_3, for binding was found to be 0.010 and 0.012 min^{-1}. Thus there was a small amount of binding in the

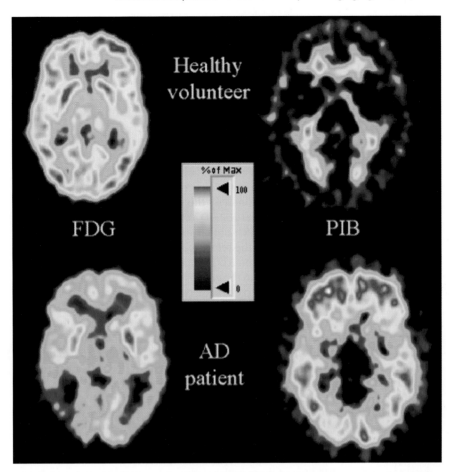

Fig. 2. PET-images of a 67year-old healthy volunteer and a 68-year-old AD patient obtained using FDG and PIB. The upper row shows normal FDG uptake (left) and lack of PIB binding (right) in the entire gray matter of the healthy volunteer. Remaining non-specific uptake is seen in the white matter. The bottom row shows a typical AD pattern with FDG (left). Areas of hypo-metabolism are present in the temporo-parieto-occipital and frontal cortices. High PIB uptake (right) is observed in the same areas.

cerebellum. We use the average value, 0.011 min^{-1}, as l_3 in the modified reference-Patlak model (Eq. 1). In cortical areas the k_2 value was found to be 0.13–0.20 min^{-1} and k_3 0.010–0.013 min^{-1}. The R-parameter was close to 1. Using Eq.1 we found that the slope was very close to k_3. In white matter with higher Aβ-density, k_2 was found to be around 0.13 min^{-1}, k_3 around 0.03 min^{-1} and R around 0.4, which means that the slope value was approximately 20% lower than the k_3-value. Based on this observations, we used the slope value from the reference-Patlak analysis as an index of the Aβ-density.

The obtained k_2- and k_3 values indicated that the half-life of the free precursor pool, $\ln2/(k_2+k_3)^{-1}$, was ON the order of 4 min in most regions. It is generally considered that after five times the biological half-life of a tracer, a steady-state between plasma and tissue has been reached. We therefore used the time interval 20-60 min for the Patlak analysis.

The metabolite analysis showed no differences between the HC and AD groups. The amount of unchanged PIB decreased rapidly and was around 60% after 5 min, 30% after 10 min and 7% after 60 min.

Figure 3a shows slopes for the PIB uptake in HC and AD groups obtained with the modified reference-Patlak method in selected regions. For each region mean value and SD are displayed. In cortical areas (parietal, frontal) the slope values in AD patients were clearly larger than in the HC group, whereas the slope values in pons and white matter were approximately the same for the two groups. In HC subjects the accumulation rate was largest in the white matter, whereas in AD patients the accumulation rate was much higher in the cortical areas than in white matter. The cerebellum constituted the reference region in both groups.

Figure 3b shows $rCMR_{glc}$ for HC and AD groups in the same regions as in Figure 3a. Again mean values and SDs within the groups are displayed. Clearly $rCMR_{glc}$ is lower in the AD patients compared to HC subjects in most regions. In accordance with the difference in Patlak slope using PIB, the largest differences in $rCMR_{glc}$ are observed in cortical areas. We observed that the relative differences in $rCMR_{glc}$ between AC and HC are in general smaller than the corresponding relative differences in PIB accumulation rate. We have also tried to use values normalized to the $rCMR_{glc}$ value in sensorimotor cortex or whole brain. With these measures the differences between AD and HC became smaller than with $rCMR_{glc}$.

Figure 4 shows the slope values using PIB plotted versus $rCMR_{glc}$ for the HC and AD groups in four different regions. Each point shows the pair of average values for one subject. Clearly the HC and AD groups were well separated in the cortical areas and almost coincide in white matter.

Two patients differ from the remaining seven, especially with respect to the accumulation rate of PIB. One of these patients showed accumulation rates similar to that found in the HC group. In the cortical areas the slope values for this patient were far below the values found in the AD group. Similarly, the rCMRglc values were within the ranges found in the HC group. The Aß level in CSF was within the reference value for AD (365 pg/ml). This patient had been on cholinesterase inhibitor treatment for four years, and his MMSE score had improved during treatment and was the highest (28). For the second outlier (80-year-old), the slope values were similar to the values found for the HC group in all regions with the exception of the parietal and frontal cortical areas. This patient showed an Aß level in CSF that was above the reference value (589 ng/ml) but showed a MMSE score of 22 and had also been on cholinesterase inhibitor treatment for four years.

The differences in slope and $rCMR_{glc}$ between the AD and HC groups in different regions are displayed in Figure 5. Clearly there is an inverse correlation between the difference in slope and the difference in $rCMR_{glc}$. Regions with large positive differences in slope tend to have large negative differences in $rCMR_{glc}$.

No clear correlation was found between slope value and MMSE or between slope value and CSF concentrations of Aβ1–42 or tau (data not shown).

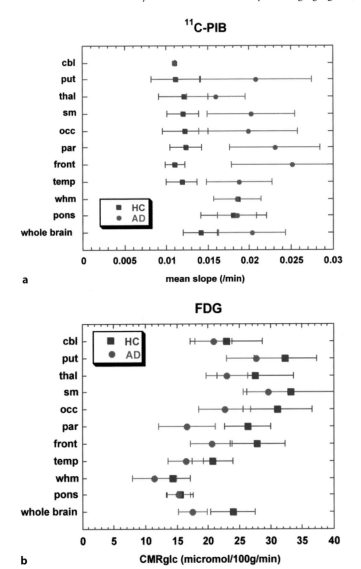

Fig. 3. Accumulation of PIB and metabolic rate in selected regions. **a)** Slope values for PIB uptake calculated with the modified reference-Patlak method. **b)** rCMR$_{glc}$. HC. n=5,;AD, n=9 are shown.

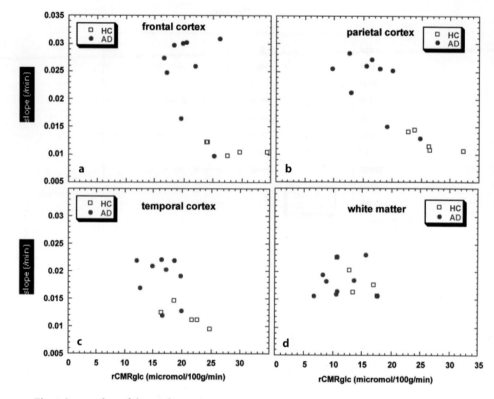

Fig. 4. Scatter plots of slope values using PIB versus rCMR$_{glc}$ in **a**) frontal cortex, **b**) parietal cortex, **c**) temporal cortex, and **d**) white matter. In the plots each point represents the pair of mean values obtained for one subject. HC, n= 5; AD, n=9

Discussion

In this study PIB was evaluated as a tracer for Aβ-density in AD brains.

PIB provided a clear discrimination between AD and HC subjects. While the absolute levels of PIB retention were approximately the same in the subcortical white matter of AD and HC subjects, the relationship between cortical areas and the white matter (WM) was opposite in AD and HC subjects. In HC subjects there was comparatively small uptake in cortical regions, leaving the WM as the predominant structure. In sharp contrast, AD cortical areas, known to contain amyloid deposits, showed preferential retention of PIB, resulting in images with high uptake in frontal and temporoparietal regions, with relatively little apparent uptake in WM. Time-activity curves show the underlying pharmacokinetic basis for the images

The experiments in the HC group with arterial blood sampling indicated that the slope value, obtained in the reference-Patlak analysis of the PIB data, was a

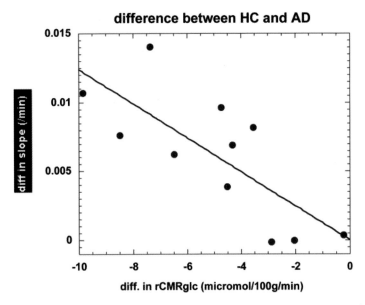

Fig. 5. Scatter plot of the difference in PIB accumulation rate between AD patients and HC versus the difference in rCMR$_{glc}$ between AD patients and HC subjects. Each point shows the average difference in slope and rCMR$_{glc}$ for one of the regions in Figure 4. The straight line is obtained by linear regression of the change in slope against change in CMR$_{glc}$. The comparison was performed between age-matched subjects. (R=0.80). HC, n=2; AD, n=9

good approximation of the accumulation rate constant k_3, which, in turn, was assumed to be proportional to the Aβ-density. In the AD group the cortical areas had slope values that were considerably higher than the corresponding values in the HC group. However, the slope is still an index of the Aβ-density. The method can be used in clinical practice where invasive arterial sampling should be avoided.

The reference region used, the cerebellum, showed a low binding of PIB. We have found that the slope values in the HC and AD groups were equal within errors in white matter and the pons. This finding was expected, because in these regions the accumulation of PIB was assumed to be an effect of non-specific binding only. Thus our results gave indirect support to the assumption of an equal accumulation rate in the cerebellum in the HC and AD groups.

The coupling between PIB and FDG metabolism was not unexpected, given the well-known decrease in frontal and temporoparietal metabolism in AD and the presence of extensive amyloid deposition in these same areas. FDG and PIB must be considered as complementary techniques, one looking directly at pathology and the other looking at metabolic dysfunction that may or may not be related to the amyloid pathology. It is assumed that pathological hallmarks of the disease, such as Aß and its plaque formation, are present in brain many years before symptoms of the disease. In spite of the correlation found between increased PIB accumulation rate and decreased glucose metabolism in AD patients compared to HC subjects, this does not mean that the metabolic deficits may be directly related to amyloid deposition. So far we have only investigated mild AD patients. It will be important to perform further studies in subjects with mild cognitive impairments (MCI) and strong heredity for AD as well as in larger groups of AD patients.

It is important to emphasize that PIB white matter labelling is apparent in controls, only because of the greater relative clearance of PIB from cortical areas. The residual white matter labelling by PIB does not appear to detract from the ability of this agent to specifically identify areas of amyloid deposition in AD.

It is interesting that there were no significant differences between the young and old controls included in this study. We hope to expand our human studies to MCI patients and to subjects at risk for AD, such as those with APP and presenilin mutations. Another of the first uses will perhaps be as an aid to the development of a variety of anti-amyloid therapeutic candidates. The carbon-11 label of PIB, with a 20-min half-life , holds several advantages for research studies. For example, it is possible to do sequential $[^{15}O]H_2O$ blood flow, PIB amyloid imaging and $[^{18}F]FDG$ glucose metabolic studies in a single imaging session. However, ^{18}F-labeling is preferable so that an imaging agent can be made widely available through local distribution networks to sites with PET cameras without an on-site cyclotron. ^{18}F-benzothiazole agents, based on the PIB structure, are in the latter stages of pre-clinical development.

References

Agdeppa ED, Kepe V, Liu J (2001) Binding characteristics of radiofluorinated 6-dialkylamino-2-naphthylethylidene derivatives as positron emission tomography imaging probes for beta-amyloid plaques in Alzheimer's disease. J Neurosci 21: RC189

Andersson JL, Thurfjell L (1997) Implementation and validation of a fully automatic system for intra- and interindividual registration of PET brain scans. J Comput Assist Tomogr 21: 136–44

Arnold SE, Hyman BT, Flory J (1991) The topographical and neuroanatomical distribution of neurofibrillary tangles and neuritic plaques in the cerebral cortex of patients with Alzheimer's disease. Cereb Cortex 1: 103–116

Bergström M, Grahnén A, Långström B (2003 PET-microdosing, a new concept with application in early clinical drug development. Eur J Clin Pharmacol 59:357–366

Blomqvist G, Engeler H, Wall A (2002). Graphical analysis of time-activity data using a references region with known irreversible binding. IX Turku PET symposium, May 25–28, Turku, Finland, p. Q01.

Braak H, Braak E (1991) Neuropathological stageing of Alzheimer-related changes. Acta Neuropathol (Berl) 82: 239–259

Dezutter NA, Landman WJ, Jager PL (2001) Evaluation of 99mTc-MAMA-chrysamine G as an in vivo probe for amyloidosis. Amyloid 8: 202–214

Engler H, Lundberg PO, Ekbom K (2003) Multitracer study with positron emission tomography in Creutzfeldt-Jakob disease. Eur J Nucl Med Mol Imaging 30: 85–95

Friedland RP, Kalaria R, Berridge M (1997) Neuroimaging of vessel amyloid in Alzheimer's disease. Ann N Y Acad Sci 826: 242–247

Gjedde A (1981) High-and low-affinity transport of D-glucose from blood to brain. J Neurochem. 36:1463–1471

Hardy J, Allsop D (1991) Amyloid deposition as the central event in the aetiology of Alzheimer's disease. Trends Pharmacol Sci 12: 383–388

Klunk WE, Jacob RF, Mason RP (1999) Quantifying amyloid beta-peptide (Abeta) aggregation using the Congo red-Abeta (CR-abeta) spectrophotometric assay. Anal Biochem 266: 66–76

Klunk WE, Wang Y, Huang GF (2001) Uncharged thioflavin-T derivatives bind to amyloid-beta protein with high affinity and readily enter the brain. Life Sci 69: 1471–1484

Wang Y, Holt DP, Huang GF, Debnath ML, Klunk WE (2003) Synthesis and evaluation of 11C-labelled 6-substituted 2-aryl benzothiazoles as amyloid imaging agents. J. Med. Chem 46:2740–2754

McKhann G, Drachman D, Folstein M (1984) Clinical diagnosis of Alzheimer's disease: report of the NINCDS-ADRDA Work Group under the auspices of Department of Health and Human Services Task Force on Alzheimer's Disease. Neurology 34: 939–944

Patlak CS, Blasberg RG (1985) Graphical evaluation of blood-to-brain transfer constants from multiple-time uptake data. Generalizations. J Cereb Blood Flow Metab 5: 584–590

Raichle ME, Martin WR, Herscovitch P (1983) Brain blood flow measured with intravenous H2(15)O. II. Implementation and validation. J Nucl Med 24: 790–798

Shoghi-Jadid K, Small GW, Agdeppa ED (2002) Localization of neurofibrillary tangles and beta-amyloid plaques in the brains of living patients with Alzheimer disease. Am J Geriatr Psychiatry 10: 24–35

Mild Cognitive Impairment (MCI): Predicting Conversion to Clinically Probable Alzheimer`s Disease with Fluoro-Deoxy-Glucose PET

J.-C. Baron[1], G. Chételat[2], B. Desgranges[2], F. Eustache[2]

Summary

Background

Optimal implementation of disease-modifying treatment for sporadic Alzheimer`s disease (AD) will require detection of patients at the pre-dementia stage. Resting-state mapping of brain glucose utilization with PET and ^{18}F-fluoro-deoxy-glucose (FDG) is sensitive to early changes in synaptic activity/density in neurodegenerative diseases such as AD. In this study, we assessed memory-impaired patients with mild cognitive impairment (MCI) and used voxel-based analysis to search for an FDG-PET profile associated with rapid conversion to AD.

Methods

We prospectively recruited 17 patients with neuropsychologically proven significant and isolated memory impairment fulfilling current criteria for amnestic MCI. We obtained resting-state [18]FDG PET and followed each patient up for a fixed period of 18 months to assess conversion to AD based on NINDS-ADRDA criteria.

Results

At the end of follow-up, seven patients had converted to AD ("converters") and the remaining ten still fulfilled criteria for MCI ("non- converters"). Using SPM99, FDG uptake in the right temporo-parietal association cortex was significantly lower in converters relative to non-converters and discriminated the two groups without overlap. FDG uptake was also lower in the converters in the posterior cingulate cortex, but discrimination was less complete and high statistical significance was not maintained after controlling for MMSE score.

---

[1] Dept. of Neurology, University of Cambridge, UK
[2] INSERM E 218-University-Cyceron, Caen, France

Hyman et al.
The Living Brain and Alzheimer's
©Springer-Verlag Berlin Heidelberg

Conclusion

This study, using an objective and comprehensive voxel-based data analysis, suggests that FDG-PET may accurately identify rapid converters.

Introduction

The ability to accurately predict progression to Alzheimer's disease at its pre-dementia stage would have major implications, especially with respect to prognosis and disease-modifying treatment (Cutler and Sramek 2001). Mild cognitive impairment (MCI), as it refers to patients with significant but isolated progressive memory impairment relative to age-matched normal subjects (i.e., "amnestic" MCI; Petersen et al. 2001), is presently the most commonly accepted reference for incipient AD because it predicts conversion to dementia more consistently than other, over-inclusive entities (Petersen et al. 2001). However, although MCI is a high-risk condition for the development of clinically probable AD, not all MCI patients rapidly progress to clinical AD (Petersen et al. 2001). The ability to reliably identify at first assessment those MCI subjects who will rapidly convert to AD would have considerable impact on design of therapeutic trials.

Changes in regional resting-state cerebral blood flow (CBF) and glucose metabolism (rCMRGlc) have been consistently reported in probable AD relative to healthy age-matched controls, with the earliest affected area being the posterior cingulate gyrus (PCG), followed by the temporo-parietal association cortex (TPACx) and hippocampal region (Baron 1998). Longitudinal studies of cognitively impaired subjects at risk of developing AD have been recently published (Celsis et al. 1997; Arnaiz et al. 2001; Johnson et al. 1998; Kogure et al. 2000; Minoshima et al. 1997; Tanaka et al. 2002; De Santi et al. 2001). Of these, only two directly compared converters to non-converters (Celsis et al. 1997; Arnaiz et al. 2001), which is the appropriate comparison if one is to address the question of what differentiates MCI patients who rapidly convert from those who do not. Although both studies reported significant TPACx hypoperfusion/hypometabolism in converters, they both assessed this region only, so whether other brain regions may perform better remained an open question. In addition, their follow-up duration was not fixed (range: 10-75 months and 1-3 years, respectively), so rapid conversion to AD was not specifically assessed. Neither study employed current criteria for defining MCI, so the relevance of their findings to amnestic MCI is unclear. Finally, they both used regions of interest (ROIs), which, in contrast to voxel-based approaches, are observer-dependent and do not assess the entire brain. Four studies compared converters to healthy controls using voxel-based techniques (Johnson et al. 1998; Kogure et al. 2000; Minoshima et al. 1997; Tanaka et al. 2002; De Santi et al. 2001) and consistently reported hypoperfusion/hypometabolism of the PCG region in the patient group, variably involving other areas in some studies. In one study that used ROIs and assessed solely the temporal lobe, significant hippocampal region hypometabolism was found in MCI subjects when contrasted to healthy controls (De Santi et al. 2001).

We prospectively recruited 19 strictly screened amnestic MCI patients, studied them with [¹⁸F]fluoro-2-deoxy-D-glucose (FDG) PET, followed them up for a pre-defined period of 18 months, and compared the initial FDG-PET profile of converters to that of non-converters using voxel-based analysis. We also compared the MCI subgroups to healthy aged controls. The results of this study have been published in part in Chételat et al. Neurolgoy, 2003, 60:1374-1377.

Methods

Subjects

According to a prospective design, right-handed amnestic MCI patients were recruited through a memory clinic, which they attended for a complaint of memory impairment (confirmed by an informant) without impairment of activities of daily living. Following comprehensive investigations, they were enrolled into this project according to the following criteria:
1. lack of neurological, medical or psychiatric disorder (including substance abuse and depression);
2. no significant focal abnormality at structural brain imaging;
3. no current medication that may affect brain function;
4. modified Hachinski ischemic score ≤ 2
5. age >55 years;
6. at least seven yrs of schooling;
7. objective episodic memory impairment, as defined by performance >1.5 SD below the mean for age-matched normal controls in at least one sub-score of Grober and Buschke's test or at Rey's figure delayed recall test; and
8. NINCDS-ADRDA criteria for probable AD (McKhann et al. 1984) not met, as documented by MMSE scores >24 and normal cognitive functions (apart from episodic memory), including executive (STROOP test), visuospatial (copy of Rey's figure), gestual praxis (imitation of four meaningless gestures, production of four symbolic gestures and four object utilization gestures), and language (writing of 12 irregular words under dictation and image naming using the DO80) functions. Patients belonging to kindred with autosomal dominant AD were excluded from the study. Each patient gave written informed consent to participate to the study, which was approved by the regional ethics committee.

For comparison, 15 unmedicated optimally healthy controls without memory complaint were also studied (see Table 1 for demographics). They were strictly screened for the absence of cerebrovascular risk factors, mental disorder, substance abuse, head trauma, significant MRI or biological abnormality, and incipient dementia.

All MCI subjects were evaluated over a period of 18 months, using the neuropsychological testing just described, to assess whether they fulfilled the NINCDS-ADRDA criteria for probable AD (McKhann et al. 1984), i.e., whether they had converted to AD. This clinical follow-up was carried out blinded to PET results. The normal controls were also reassessed 18 months after the PET study.

Table 1. Subjects' demographics (mean ± SD).

	Controls	MCI	Non-converters	Converters
N	15	17	10	7
Age (years)	62.3 ± 9.3	69.9 ± 6.5 [a]	67.8 ± 7	73 ± 5.1 [a]
Female/Male	9 / 6	9 / 8	5 /5	4 / 3
MMSE (/30)	-	27.2 ± 1.3	27.8 ± 1.2	26.3 ± 1 [c]

[a] Signifficantly different from controls (p<0.05; two-sample t test)
[b] MMSE: Mini-Mental State Examination.
[c] Significantly different from non-converters (p <0.05, two-sample t-test)

PET procedure

At entry, each subject underwent an FDG-PET study using the high-resolution PET device ECAT Exact HR+ with isotropic resolution of 4.6 x 4.2 x 4.2 mm (FOV = 158 mm). The subjects fasted for at least four hours before scanning. The head was positioned on a headrest according to the cantho-meatal line and gently restrained with straps. FDG uptake was measured in the resting condition, with eyes closed, in a quiet and dark environment. A catheter was introduced in a vein of the arm to inject the radiotracer. Following ^{68}Ga transmission scans, 3-5 mCi of ^{18}FDG were injected as a bolus at time 0, and a 10-min PET data acquisition scan was commenced 50 min post-injection. Sixty-three planes were acquired with septa out ("volume acquisition"), using a voxel size of 2.2 x 2.2 x 2.43 mm (x y z). During PET data acquisition, head motion was continuously monitored with laser beams projected onto ink marks drawn over the forehead skin.

Image handling and transformation

Using statistical parametric mapping (SPM-99) (Wellcome Dept. of Cognitive Neurology, London, UK), the PET data were subjected to an affine and non-linear spatial normalization into standard Talairach and Tournoux's space, using the MNI PET template of SPM-99, and a reslicing of 2 x 2 x 2 mm. This spatially normalized set was then smoothed with a 14-mm isotropic Gaussian filter to blur individual variations in gyral anatomy and to increase the signal-to-noise ratio.

Statistical analysis

The PET data of converters were compared to that of non-converters using the "compare-populations: 1 scan/subject (two sample t-test)" routine of SPM-99. The "proportional scaling" routine was used to control for individual variation in global FDG uptake; these normalized data will be referred to as "normalized regional activity" in what follows. To minimize "edge effects," only those voxels with values above 80% of the mean for the whole brain were selected for the statistical analysis; using an in-house routine and the Analyze software, we verified that, with this threshold, the relevant brain parenchyma, including the hippocampal region, was encompassed in the SPM analysis. SPM maps of the comparison of normalized regional activity between converters and non-converters were thresholded at Z>3.09; only decreases were assessed, Because of the inconsistencies in the literature (see Introduction), we had no strong a priori hypothesis about which area, if any, would differentiate converters from non-converters, so a peak was considered statistically significant if it reached the stringent statistical cut-off of p<0.05, cluster-level corrected; the findings with p< 0.001 [uncorrected but with (k>100 voxels) cluster extent cut-off] will also be reported as exploratory. Anatomical localization was according to both the MRI template of SPM99 and Talairach's Atlas, using M. Brett's set of linear transformations (see: www.mrc-cbu.cam.ac.uk/Imaging/mnispace.html). All coordinates presented in this article are Talairach's.

Subsequently, using SPM99, the plot of fitted and adjusted normalized regional activity value in each significant peak was obtained, and the accuracy of these values to discriminate the two MCI sub-groups was determined in the classical way by calculating the number of patients correctly classified divided by the total number of patients (x 100).

For the sake of completeness, we also compared the PET data of each MCI sub-group, as well as of the whole group, to the data of the healthy aged controls using SPM99 and the above procedure. For this analysis, and based on prior literature (see Introduction), we had a strong a priori hypothesis that the posterior cingulate/precuneus region would be significantly reduced in MCI patients relative to normal controls, so a cut-off of p<0.005 was considered significant for this area only. Results with less stringent cut-offs will also be reported for heuristic purposes. Because there was a significant difference in age between converters and controls, and between the whole MCI group and controls (see Table 1), age was added as a "nuisance variable" in the SPM comparisons.

Results

Of the 19 patients, one refused repeated cognitive testing and another turned out to have depression. Thus, 17 patients were eligible for this analysis. At completion of follow-up, seven patients met NINCDS-ADRDA for probable AD, whereas the remaining ten patients still fulfilled the operational criteria for MCI. The two sub-groups did not significantly differ in age but converters had slightly but significantly lower entry MMSE scores than nonconverters (Table 1). None of the 15 healthy aged controls met NINCDS-ADRDA for probable AD at the end of the follow-up period.

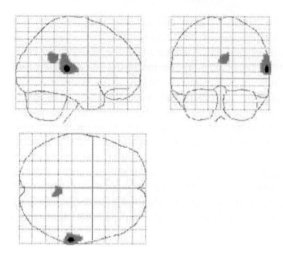

Fig. 1. SPM99 "glass brain" maps showing the significant decreases (p<0.001, uncorrected; cluster extent k>100 voxels) in normalized regional activity in converters (n=7) as compared to non-converters (N=10), showing right temporo-parietal and posterior cingulate clusters.

Converters vs. non-converters (Fig. 1)

At the p<0.05 cluster-level corrected cut-off, SPM revealed a single peak of decrease in normalized regional activity in the posterior part of the right superior temporal gyrus (63 –27 12, x y z; p, cluster-level corrected = 0.02; Z = 4.82; cluster extent K = 470), but encroaching upon the neighboring inferior parietal cortex. At the more liberal p<0.001 level, there was one additional peak in the right PCG (6 –45 26, x y z; Z = 3.68; K = 133), straddling the left homologous area. Scatter plots showed that in the right temporo-parietal peak, discrimination between the two sub-groups was complete, without overlap (accuracy=100%), whereas in the PCG peak, one subject was misclassified (accuracy: 94%). To control for the significant difference in MMSE scores between converters and non-converters, the SPM analysis was reprocessed with the MMSE score as a "nuisance variable." The right temporo-parietal peak was recovered with unchanged coordinates and statistical significance (63 –29 12, x y z; p, cluster-level corrected = 0.015; Z = 4.48; K = 536); the PCG peak was recovered only at a cut-off of p<0.005, uncorrected (8 –47 26, x y z; Z = 2.69; K = 109).

Comparisons with Controls

Whole MCI group (Fig. 2). At the p < 0.005 (uncorrected) threshold, there was a single peak of decrease, located in the precuneus/PCG (14 –60 34, x y z; p, uncorrected = 0.002; Z = 2.84; K = 124).

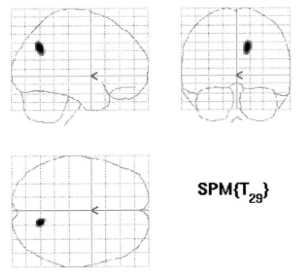

Fig. 2. SPM99 "glass brain" maps showing the significant decreases (p<0.005, uncorrected; adjusted for age) in normalized regional activity in the whole MCI group (n=17) as compared to healthy controls (N=15), showing a single right posterior cingulate cluster.

Non-converters. There was no finding for this comparison, even at the very liberal cut-off of p < 0.01.

Converters (Fig. 3). There was a single peak of significant decrease in the right PCG (10 –58 36, x y z; p=0.029, cluster-level corrected; $Z = 4.32$; K = 395), straddling the left PCG. At the p < 0.005 (uncorrected) cut-off, there was another peak in the right superior temporal gyrus, very close to the peak found in the converters vs non-converters comparison (61 –34 16, x y z; p, uncorrected = 0.002; $Z = 2.97$; K = 76).

Discussion

This is the first study of MCI that prospectively assesses the difference in initial metabolic profile between converters and non-converters by means of voxel-based analysis. We found that MCI patients who rapidly converted to probable AD had highly significantly lower initial FDG uptake in the right temporo-parietal cortex than did those who did not convert, without individual overlap, whereas the PCG afforded less significant and less complete differentiation.

The 18-month follow-up period used in this study was prospectively chosen as being meaningful both clinically and for future trials of disease-modifying agents. The rate of conversion to AD (around 25% per year) was well within reported ranges for amnestic MCI (Petersen et al. 2001). Despite wide individual overlap,

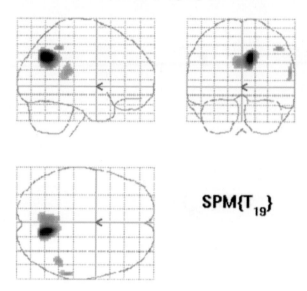

SPM{T$_{19}$}

Fig. 3. SPM99 "glass brain" maps showing the significant decreases (p<0.005, uncorrected; adjusted for age) in normalized regional activity in the converters (n=7) as compared to healthy controls (N=15), showing bilateral posterior cingulate and right temporo-parietal clusters.

there was a statistically significant difference in MMSE score at entry between the two sub-groups, consistent with earlier studies that found lower memory performance is associated with higher risk of conversion (Small et al. 1997; Visser et al. 2000). Post-hoc SPM reprocessing controlling for this potential confounder recovered the same right temporo-parietal area with unchanged significance; in contrast, the posterior cingulate region lost its discriminating value.

The area found to best discriminate converters from non-converters is the posterior part of the superior temporal gyrus (Brodmann`s area 42), encroaching upon the neighboring planum temporale and supramarginal gyrus. This region of the TPACx is part of the typical hypometabolic profile of mild AD (Baron 1998), and hypometabolism in this area relative to healthy controls has been documented in non-demented subjects at risk of developing AD, such as ApoE4 carriers (Small et al. 2000; Reiman et al. 1996) and asymptomatic carriers of mutations for autosomal dominant AD (Johnson et al. 2001; Kennedy et al. 1995)]. Furthermore, our finding is consistent with two earlier, similar studies that directly compared converters to non-converters (Celsis et al. 1997; Arnaiz et al. 2001), both of which reported metabolic alterations (asymmetry or decrease) in the TPACx. However, both studies had several methodological limitations (see Introduction), and the accuracy of the metabolic alterations found in predicting conversion was incomplete in both. Moreover, only the TPACx was assessed in these two studies; the question of whether other brain regions might have done a better job was not considered. Our study is the first to use a voxel-based image analysis, and the results show that the right temporo-parietal region was able to identify, among amnestic MCI patients, those who rapidly converted to clinically probable AD.

That the temporo-parietal difference concerned the right side only is intriguing. However, it is consistent with the study of Celsis et al., (1997) which found that four of the five converters had predominant right-sided hypoperfusion. Although only the left temporo-parietal area was involved in Arnaiz et al. (2001), patients in this study were selected according to significant impairment in any area of cognition, as compared to amnesia in our study. Even with a threshold of p<0.01, we found no difference between the two MCI subgroups in the left TPACx (data not shown). This finding therefore suggests early right temporo-parietal functional alteration in AD, subtending non-mnemonic (Shapleske et al. 1999; Karnath 2001) alterations that become clinically eloquent when converting to dementia. Alternatively, subjects with left impairment (likely to be more clinically eloquent) may already qualify for clinically probable AD at the same disease stage when subjects with right impairment are still clinically judged as MCI, an idea supported by our MRI study showing that gray matter loss in AD relative to MCI is considerably greater in the left than right TPACx (Chételat et al. 2002).

In our study, PCG hypometabolism in converters was highly significant when compared to normal controls, and marginally significant when compared to non-converters. These findings are consistent with the literature. Relative to healthy controls, hypometabolism of the PCG has been previously documented in converters (Johnson et al. 1998; Kogure et al. 2000; Minoshima et al. 1997; Tanaka et al. 2002), as well as in ApoE4 (Small et al. 2000; Reiman et al. 1996) and familial AD mutation carriers (Johnson et al. 2001; Kennedy et al. 1995). Our finding that the PCG essentially lost all significance when controlling for MMSE scores suggests that hypometabolism in this region is related more strictly to the degree of global cognitive alteration than to the risk of rapid conversion to AD, which is corroborated by the direct comparison to non-converters. This para-limbic region is thought to be involved in episodic memory, as shown by 1) permanent amnesia after vascular damage limited to this region (Valenstein et al. 1987), 2) consistent hypometabolism of this region in patients with permanent non-progressive amnesia (Aupée et al. 2001), and 3) consistent activation of this region in episodic memory tasks in normal subjects (Cabeza and Nyberg 2000). As MCI is characterized by episodic memory impairment, our finding that the PCG was less predictive of conversion to AD than the temporo-parietal area would be consistent with its cognitive role.

How do our findings relate to current knowledge of the topographic progression of *tau* histopathological lesions? According to Braak`s hierarchical model of *tau* pathology (Braak and Braak 1996), the hippocampal area is the first to be affected. However, at this stage, the cognitive status may still be unaltered, whereas at advanced stages, when the lesions involve the superior temporal, inferior parietal and prefrontal polymodal association areas, almost all subjects are demented (Delacourte et al. 1999; Mitchell et al. 2002). Our finding that FDG uptake in the TPACx accurately predicted progression to dementia at a stage when there was pure memory impairment would appear to conflict with Braak`s model. Two mechanisms in converters may account for this apparent paradox: 1) partial functional compensation for local histopathological damage or 2) more likely, disrupted biochemistry/neurotransmission (shortly) preceding the development of *tau* pathology and attending clinical expression.

The lack of significant difference in FDG uptake in the hippocampal region between converters and non-converters in this study would be consistent with Braak`s model that predicts that MCI patients all have medial temporal lesions (Braak and Braak 1996; Delacourte et al. 1999; Mitchell et al. 2002). Nevertheless, converters have significantly reduced hippocampal region size as compared to non-converters [see Chételat and Baron 2003 for review], suggesting a difference in degree of damage. In our study, the hippocampal region was significantly hypometabolic relative to normal aged controls in neither the whole MCI group nor any of the two sub-groups. Apart from methodological issues (Mega et al. 2000), this discrepancy may reflect some functional/synaptic compensation for the neuronal damage (Matsuda et al. 2002). Further investigations are needed to test this hypothesis. De Santi et al. (2001) recently reported significantly lower entorhinal cortex, but not temporal neocortex, glucose metabolism in MCI patients relative to aged normals. However, they used ROIs, and the accuracy of entorhinal cortex CMRGlc in discriminating MCI from controls was only 81%.

Our study suggests that it is possible, using FDG-PET, to accurately identify those MCI patients who are soon to convert to clinically probable AD. Pending replication in an independent sample, our findings may have implications for trials of disease-modifying agents.

Acknowledgments

We are indebted to Drs. F. Viader, V. de la Sayette, D. Hannequin, F. Le Doze, S. Schaeffer and B. Dupuy for referring their patients, Dr C.Godeau for recruiting some of the volunteers, C. Lalevee for neuropsychological assessment, and the staff of Cyceron for performing the PET studies. This project was supported by INSERM U320, PHRC (Ministère de la Santé) and Association France Alzheimer.

References

Arnaiz E, Jelic V, Almkvist O, Wahlund LO, Winblad B, Valind S, Nordberg A (2001) Impaired cerebral glucose metabolism and cognitive functioning predict deterioration in mild cognitive impairment. Neuro Report 12:851–855

Aupée AM, Desgranges B, Eustache F, Lalevee C, de la Sayette V, Viader F, Baron JC (2001) Voxel-based mapping of brain hypometabolism in permanent amnesia with PET. Neuro Image 13:1164–1173

Baron JC (1998) Démences et troubles de la mémoire d'origine dégénérative: Apport de l'imagerie fonctionnelle. Rev Neurol (Paris) 154:122–130

Braak H, Braak E (1996) Evolution of the neuropathology of Alzheimer`s disease. Acta Neurol Scand165:3–12

Cabeza R, Nyberg L (2000) Imaging cognition II: An empirical review of 275 PET and fMRI studies. J Cogn Neurosci 12:1–47

Celsis P, Agniel A, Cardebat D, Demonet JF, Ousset PJ, Puel M (1997) Age related cognitive decline: a clinical entity? A longitudinal study of cerebral blood flow and memory performance. J Neurol Neurosurg Psychiat 62:601–608

Chételat G, Desgranges B, de la Sayette V, Viader F, Eustache F, Baron J-C (2002) Mapping gray matter loss with voxel-based morphometry in mild cognitive impairment. NeuroReport 13: 1939–1943

Chételat G., Baron J-C (2003) Early diagnosis of Alzheimer`s disease: contribution of structural imaging. NeuroImage 18:525–541

Cutler NR, Sramek JJ (2001) Review of the next generation of Alzheimer's disease therapeutics: challenges for drug development. Prog Neuropsychopharmacol Biol Psychiat 25:27–57

Delacourte A, David JP, Sergeant N, Buee L, Wattez A, Vermersch P, Ghozali F, Fallet-Bianco C, Pasquier F, Lebert F, Petit H, Di Menza C (1999) The biochemical pathway of neurofibrillary degeneration in aging and Alzheimer's disease. Neurology 52:1158–1165

De Santi S, de Leon MJ, Rusinek H, Convit A, Tarshish CY, Roche A, Tsui WH, Kandil E, Boppana M, Daisley K, Wang GJ, Schlyer D, Fowler J (2001) Hippocampal formation glucose metabolism and volume losses in MCI and AD. Neurobiol Aging 22:529–539

Johnson KA, Jones K, Holman BL, Becker JA, Spiers PA, Satlin A, Albert MS. (1998) Preclinical prediction of Alzheimer's disease using SPECT. Neurology 50:1563–1571

Johnson KA, Lopera F, Jones K, Becker A, Sperling R, Hilson J, Londono J, Siegert I, Arcos M, Moreno S, Madrigal L, Ossa J, Pineda N, Ardila A, Roselli M, Albert MS, Kosik KS, Rios A (2001) Presenilin-1-associated abnormalities in regional cerebral perfusion. Neurology 56:1545–1551

Karnath HO (2001) New insights into the functions of the superior temporal cortex. Nature Rev Neurosci 2:568–576

Kennedy AM, Newman SK, Frackowiak RS, Cunningham VJ, Roques P, Stevens J, Neary D, Bruton CJ, Warrington EK, Rossor MN (1995) Deficits in cerebral glucose metabolism demonstrated by positron emission tomography in individuals at risk of familial Alzheimer's disease. Neurosci Lett 186:17–20

Kogure D, Matsuda H, Ohnishi T, Asada T, Uno M, Kunihiro T, Nakano S, Takasaki M (2000) Longitudinal evaluation of early Alzheimer's disease using brain perfusion SPECT. J Nucl Med 41:1155–1162

Matsuda H, Kitayama N, Ohnishi T, Asada T, Nakano S, Sakamoto S, Imabayashi E, Katoh A (2002) Longitudinal evaluation of both morphologic and functional changes in the same individuals with Alzheimer's disease. J Nucl Med 43:304–311

McKhann G, Drachman D, Folstein M, Katzman R, Price D, Stadlan EM (1984) Clinical diagnosis of Alzheimer's disease: report of the NINCDS-ADRDA Work Group under the auspices of Department of Health and Human Services Task Force on Alzheimer's Disease. Neurology 34:939–944

Mega MS, Thompson PM, Toga AW, Cummings JL (2000) Brain mapping in dementia. In: Mazziotta JC, Toga AW, Frackowiak RSJ (eds) Brain mapping: the disorders. Academic Press, San Diego, pp 217–239

Minoshima S, Giordani B, Berent S, Frey KA, Foster NL, Kuhl DE (1997) Metabolic reduction in the posterior cingulate cortex in very early Alzheimer's disease. Ann Neurol 42:85–94

Mitchell TW, Mufson EJ, Schneider JA, Cochran EJ, Nissanov J, Han LY, Bienias JL, Lee VM, Trojanowski JQ, Bennett DA, Arnold SE (2002) Parahippocampal Tau pathology in healthy aging, mild cognitive impairment, and early Alzheimer's disease. Ann Neurol 51:182–189

Petersen RC, Doody R, Kurz A, Mohs RC, Morris JC, Rabins PV, Ritchie K, Rossor M, Thal L, Winblad B (2001) Current concepts in mild cognitive impairment. Arch Neurol 58:1985–1992

Reiman EM, Caselli RJ, Yun LS, Chen K, Bandy D, Minoshima S, Thibodeau SN, Osborne D (1996) Preclinical evidence of Alzheimer's disease in persons homozygous for the epsilon 4 allele for apolipoprotein E. N Engl J Med 334:752–758

Shapleske J, Rossell SL, Woodruff PW, David AS (1999) The planum temporale: a systematic, quantitative review of its structural, functional and clinical significance. Brain Res Brain Res Rev 29:26–49

Small BJ, Viitanen M, Backman L (1997) Mini-Mental State Examination item scores as predictors of Alzheimer's disease: incidence data from the Kungsholmen Project, Stockholm. J Gerontol A Biol Sci Med Sci 52:299–304

Small GW, Ercoli LM, Silverman DH, Huang SC, Komo S, Bookheimer SY, Lavretsky H, Miller K, Siddarth P, Rasgon NL, Mazziotta JC, Saxena S, Wu HM, Mega MS, Cummings JL, Saunders AM, Pericak-Vance MA, Roses AD, Barrio JR, Phelps ME (2000) Cerebral metabolic and cognitive decline in persons at genetic risk for Alzheimer's disease. Proc Natl Acad Sci USA 97:6037–6042

Tanaka M, Fukuyama H, Yamauchi H, Narita M, Natabame H, Yokode M, Fujimoto N, Kita T, Murakami M (2002) Regional cerebral blood flow abnormalities in nondemented patients with memory impairment. J Neuroimaging 12:112–118

Valenstein E, Bowers D, Verfaellie M, Heilman KM, Day A, Watson RT (1987) Retrosplenial amnesia. Brain 110:1631–1646

Visser PJ, Verhey FR, Ponds RW, Cruts M, Van Broeckhoven CL, Jolles J (2000) Course of objective memory impairment in non-demented subjects attending a memory clinic and predictors of outcome. Int J Geriatr Psychiat 15:363–372

Positron Emission Tomography and Magnetic Resonance Imaging in the Study of Cognitively Normal Persons at Differential Genetic Risk for Alzheimer's Dementia

Eric M. Reiman[1], Richard J. Caselli[2], Kewei Chen[3], and Gene E. Alexander[4]

Summary

Patients with Alzheimer's dementia (AD) have characteristic and progressive reductions in fluorodeoxyglucose positron emission tomography (PET) measurements of the cerebral metabolic rate for glucose and in magnetic resonance imaging (MRI) measurements of hippocampal and whole brain volume. We have been using PET and MRI to characterize and compare PET and MRI measurements in cognitively normal persons with two copies, one copy, and no copies of the apolipoprotein E ε4 allele, a common AD susceptibility gene. This article reviews and updates our previously published PET and MRI findings. It indicates how these imaging techniques could be used to help bridge existing gaps between ante-mortem and post-mortem studies of AD, non-demented persons at risk for AD, and relevant animal models. It suggests how they could provide clues about the earliest brain changes involved in the pathogenesis of AD and assist in the identification of new targets for the discovery of drugs in the treatment and prevention of this disorder. Finally, it describes a brain imaging strategy for the efficient evaluation of prevention therapies, without having to conduct studies in thousands of research subjects, restrict these studies to those who are older or are already symptomatic, or wait many years to determine whether or when treated individuals develop mild cognitive impairment or AD.

Introduction

Alzheimer's dementia (AD) is a devastating illness and a rapidly growing public health problem. Clinically, this disorder is characterized by a gradual and progressive decline in memory and other cognitive functions, including language skills, the recognition of faces and objects, the performance of routine tasks, and executive functions, and it is frequently associated with other distressing and disabling behavioral problems (McKhann et al. 1984; American Psychiatric Association

[1] Department of Psychiatry, University of Arizona (EMR), [2] Department of Neurology, Mayo Clinic Scottsdale (RJC), [3] Department of Mathematics (KC) and [4] Psychology (GEA), Arizona State University, Good Samaritan Positron Emission Tomography Center (EMR, KC), and Arizona Alzheimer's Disease Consortium (EMR, RJC, GEA, KC), 1111 East McDowell Road, Phoenix, AZ 85006

Hyman et al.
The Living Brain and Alzheimer's
©Springer-Verlag Berlin Heidelberg

1994; Reiman et al. 1999). Histopathological features of AD include neuritic and diffuse plaques (in which the major constituent is the β-amyloid protein), neurofibrillary tangles (in which the major constituent is the hyperphosphorylated form of the microtubule-associated protein tau), and the loss of neurons and synapses (Terry et al. 1999). In addition to its effects on patients, AD places a terrible burden on the family; indeed, about half of the affected persons' primary caregivers become clinically depressed (Cohen and Eisdorfer 1988). According to one community survey, AD afflicts about 10% of those over the age of 65 and almost half of those over the age of 85 (Evans et al. 1989). As the population grows older, the prevalence and cost of AD is expected to increase dramatically (Katzman and Kawas 1994). For example, by 2050 the prevalence of AD in the United States has been projected to quadruple (from about 4 to 16 million cases, even without assuming an increase in an affected person's life expectancy), and the cost of caring for patients will quadruple (from about 190 to 750 million dollars per year, even without any adjustment for inflation) (Reiman et al. 2001a). An AD prevention therapy is urgently needed to avert an overwhelming public health problem.

Scientific progress has raised the hope of identifying treatments to halt the progression and prevent the onset of AD (Reiman et al. 2001b). This progress includes 1) the discovery of genetic mutations and of at least one susceptibility gene that account for many cases of AD; 2) the characterization of other AD risk factors and pathogenic molecular events that could be targeted by potential treatments; 3) the development and use of improved research methods (e.g., in the fields of genomics and proteomics) for the identification of new therapeutic targets; 4) the development of promising animal models, including transgenic mice containing one or more AD genes, which may help clarify disease mechanisms and screen candidate treatments; 5) suggestive evidence that several available interventions (e.g., anti-inflammatory medications, statins, vitamin E, folic acid, and Ginkgo biloba), which may be associated with a lower risk and later onset of AD; 6) the discovery of medications which at least modestly attenuate AD symptoms (e.g., several acetylcholinesterase inhibitors and the N-methyl-D-aspartate [NMDA] inhibitor memantine); and 7) the development of other potentially disease-modifying investigational treatments (e.g., histopathological immunization and sequestration therapies, drugs that inhibit the production, aggregation, and neurotoxic sequelae of Aβ, drugs that inhibit the hyperphosphorylation of tau, and drugs that protect neurons against oxidative, inflammatory, excitatory, and other potentially toxic events).

Even if a prevention therapy is only modestly helpful, it could provide an extraordinary public health benefit. For instance, a therapy that delays the mean onset of AD by only five years might reduce the number of cases by half (Khachaturian 1992). Unfortunately, it would require thousands of volunteers, many years, and great expense to determine whether or when cognitively normal persons treated with a candidate primary prevention therapy develop cognitive impairment and AD. One way to reduce the samples and time required to assess the efficacy of an AD prevention therapy is to conduct a clinical trial in patients with mild cognitive impairment (MCI), who may have a 10-15% rate of conversion to probable AD and commonly have histopathological features of AD at autopsy (Petersen et al. 1999; Morris et al. 2001). Randomized, placebo-controlled clinical trials in patients with MCI could thus help establish the efficacy of putative "secondary prevention" therapies. Using clinical outcome measures, the only practical way to establish the efficacy of a "primary prevention" therapy has been to restrict the randomized, placebo-controlled study to subjects in advanced age groups – a strategy that still requires extremely large samples, a study duration of several years, and significant cost. While these strategies are likely to play significant roles in the identification of effective prevention therapies, it remains possible that subjects will require treatment at a younger age or at an even earlier stage of underlying disease for a candidate prevention therapy to exert its most beneficial effects. Researchers in academics and industry recognize the value of developing putative primary prevention therapies, and they are placing an increasing emphasis on the earliest possible detection of the brain changes associated with the predisposition to this disorder. A new paradigm is needed to reduce the subject samples, time, and cost required to establish the efficacy of putative primary prevention therapies, encourage industry and government agencies to sponsor the required trials, and prevent this growing problem without losing a generation along the way.

With this goal in mind, we have been using fluorodeoxyglucose (FDG) positron emission tomography (PET) and volumetric magnetic resonance imaging (MRI) to detect and track the changes in brain function and structure that precede the onset of symptoms in cognitively normal persons carrying two copies, one copy, and no copies of the apolipoprotein E (APOE) ε4 allele, a common susceptibility gene that accounts for many cases of late-onset AD. In this review article, we provide background information from relevant genetic and brain imaging studies of AD, we review our published brain imaging studies of cognitively normal persons at differential genetic risk for AD and findings presented in recent abstracts, we suggest new applications to the study of promising animal models (e.g., transgenic mice) and the post-mortem human brain, and we describe our strategy for using FDG PET (and volumetric MRI) in the efficient evaluation of prevention therapies.

The APOE ε4 Allele:
A Common AD Susceptibility Gene

Suggested risk factors for AD include older age, female gender, lower educational level, a history of head trauma, cardiovascular disease, higher cholesterol and homocysteine levels, lower serum folate levels, a reported family history of AD; trisomy 21 (Down's syndrome), at least 12 missense mutations of the amyloid precursor peptide (APP) gene on chromosome 21, at least 92 missense mutations of the presenilin 1 (PS1) gene on chromosome 14, at least 8 missense mutations of the presenilin 2 (PS2) gene on chromosome 1, candidate susceptibility loci on chromosomes 10 and 12, and the APOE ε4 allele on chromosome 19 (http://molgen-www.uia.ac.be/ADMutations) (Reiman et al. 2001b; Seshadri et al. 2002; Snowdon et al. 2000). Whereas some of these risk factors are well established (e.g., age, AD mutations, and the ε4 allele), others are less well supported and require further investigation (e.g., genetic loci on chromosomes 10 and 12). The APP, PS1, and

PS2 mutations appear to account for about 70% of cases "early onset AD" (with onset typically before the age of 60) and they cause forms of the disorder characterized by autosomal dominant inheritance with age-dependent penetrance. Whereas these "AD genes" account for fewer than 5% of all AD cases, researchers have identified at least one "AD susceptibility gene," the APOE ε4 allele, that accounts for many cases of late-onset AD (with onset typically after the age of 60) with or without a reported family history of the disorder (Strittmatter et al. 1993; Saunders et al. 1993; Corder et al. 1993; Farrer et al. 1997). While the APOE ε4 is not associated with an elevation in plasma levels of Aβ, the APOE E4 isoform has been shown to be a pathological chaperone for the aggregation of Aβ (Wisniewski et al. 1994); conversely, it has been suggested that the APOE isoforms associated with a lower risk of AD may inhibit Aβ-induced cytotoxicity (Miyata and Smith 1996) and may bind to tau, preventing hyperphosphorylation (Strittmatter et al. 1994). In addition, APOE isoforms may influence the risk of AD through their differential effects on the distribution and metabolism of cholesterol (Mahley 1988) or other mechanisms that remain to be discovered.

Next to age, the APOE ε4 allele is the best-established risk factor for late-onset AD, and thus, it is especially relevant to our human brain imaging studies. The APOE gene has three major alleles: ε2, ε3, and ε4 (Mahley 1988). In comparison with the ε3 allele (the most common variant), the ε4 allele is associated with a higher risk of AD and a younger age at dementia onset, whereas the ε2 allele may be associated with a lower risk of AD and an older age at dementia onset (Strittmatter et al. 1993; Saunders et al. 1993; Corder et al. 1993; Farrer et al. 1997; Corder et al. 1994). In one of the original case-control studies, individuals with no copies of the ε4 allele had a 20% risk of AD and a median age of 84 at dementia onset, those with one copy of the ε4, which is found in about 24% of the population (Mahley 1988) had a 47% risk of AD and a median age of 76 at dementia onset, and those with two copies of the ε4 allele [the ε4/ε4 genotype, found in 2–3% of the population (Mahley 1988)] had a 91% risk of AD by 80 years and a mean age of 68 at dementia onset (Corder et al. 1993). In another study, 100% of ε4 carriers with cognitive loss had neuritic plaques at autopsy (Saunders et al. 1996). In a related study, 23% of their AD cases were attributed to absence of the ε2 allele and another 65% of their cases were attributed to the presence of one or more copies of the ε4 allele (Corder et al. 1994). Case-control studies in numerous clinical, neuropathological, and community studies have confirmed the association between the ε4 allele and AD. Farrer et al. (1997) conducted a worldwide meta-analysis of data from 5930 patients with probable or autopsy-confirmed AD and 8607 controls from various ethnic and racial backgrounds. In comparison with persons with the genotype ε3/ε3, the risk of AD was significantly increased in genotypes ε2/ε4 (odds ratio [OR]=2.6), ε3/ε4 (OR=3.2), and ε4/ε4 (OR=14.9), and the risk of AD was significantly decreased in genotypes ε2/ε3 (OR=0.6), and ε2/ε2 (OR=0.6). Community-based, prospective studies promise to better characterize the absolute risk of AD in persons with each APOE genotype.

In a longitudinal brain imaging study, we have been capitalizing on the study of ε4 homozygotes, ε4 heterozygotes (all with the ε3/ε4 genotype), and ε4 noncarriers who were initially late middle-aged (i.e., younger than the suggested median onset of AD), cognitively normal, and individually matched for their gender, age, and educational level. Since individuals with the ε4/ε4 genotype have an especially high risk of AD, the study of this subject group is intended to optimize our power to characterize the brain and behavioral changes that precede the onset of cognitive impairment and eventually relate these changes to the subsequent onset of MCI and AD. Since individuals with the ε3/ε4 genotype have an increased risk of AD and comprise about 20-23% of the population (Mahley 1988), the study of this subject group is intended to extend our findings to a larger segment of the population and increase the number of individuals who would be eligible to participate in future clinical trials of putative primary prevention therapies. The study of ε4 noncarriers who are individually matched for gender, age, and educational level could optimize the power to characterize the brain and behavioral changes associated with normal aging and permit us to distinguish them from those age-related changes preferentially related to the presence of the ε4 allele and the subsequent onset of AD. As other risk factors are confirmed, it should be possible to extend our brain imaging paradigm and findings to the study of cognitively normal persons who are at differential risk for AD independent of (and in conjunction with) their APOE genotype.

PET In the Study of AD

FDG PET, which provides measurements of the cerebral metabolic rate for glucose (CMRgl), is the most extensively used functional brain imaging technique in the study, early detection, and tracking of AD. FDG PET reveals characteristic abnormalities in patients with AD, including abnormally low posterior cingulate, parietal, and temporal CMRgl, abnormally low prefrontal and whole brain CMRgl in more severely affected patients, and a progressive decline in these and other measurements over time (de Leon et al. 1983; Foster et al. 1983; Duara et al. 1986; Jagust et al. 1988; Haxby et al. 1990; McGeer et al. 1990; Smith et al. 1992; Minoshima et al. 1994,1995; Mielke et al. 1994; Mega et al. 1997; Ibanez et al. 1998; Hoffman et al. 2000; Silverman et al. 2001; Alexander et al. 2002a). These abnormalities, which are correlated with dementia severity and predict subsequent clinical decline and the histopathological diagnosis of AD (Jagust et al. 1988; Haxby et al. 1990; McGeer et al. 1990; Smith et al. 1992; Mielke et al. 1994; Mega et al. 1997; Hoffman et al. 2000; Silverman et al. 2001), could be related to a reduction in the activity or density of terminal neuronal fields or perisynaptic glial cells that innervate these regions (Schwartz et al. 1979; Meguro et al. 1999; Magistretti and Pellerin 1996), a metabolic dysfunction (Magistretti and Pellerin 1996; Piert et al. 1996; Mark et al. 1997), or a combination of these factors. They do not appear to be solely attributable to the combined effects of atrophy and partial-volume averaging (Ibanez et al. 1998).

We recently used FDG PET and a commonly used brain mapping algorithm (SPM99) to compare regional CMRgl in 14 patients with probable AD and 34 normal control subjects, to compute 1-year CMRgl declines in the patients, and to estimate the number of patients needed to detect a significant effect of a candidate treatment in a one-year, double-blind, placebo-controlled clinical trial (Alexander et al. 2001). As in previous studies, the patients with probable AD had significantly lower measurements of CMRgl than the normal control subjects bilaterally in regions of the parietal, temporal, occipital, frontal, and posterior cingulate cortex. One year later, the patients with AD had significant CMRgl declines in each of these locations and in the whole brain. The average annual rate of CMRgl decline in these regions (in absolute measurements of mg/min/100 g) varied between 6 and 11%, and the CMRgl reductions were so extensive that efforts to normalize the data for the variation in absolute measurements, using either the whole brain or pons as a reference region, led to an underestimation of these declines. The number of patients with probable AD needed in each arm of a placebo-controlled study to detect different treatment effects with 80% power is noted in Table 1. The estimated power of PET to detect an effect of a putative treatment in patients with AD was significantly greater than the clinical ratings or neuropsychological test scores used in this study and roughly comparable to previously reported power estimates using MRI.

Studies from our group in Arizona and Gary Small's group in California indicate that these abnormalities can be detected prior to the onset of dementia (Reiman et al. 1996, 2001a,b; Small et al. 1995; Small et al. 2000). As described in another section, we have been studying cognitively normal ε4 homozygotes, heterozygotes, and noncarriers, 47-68 years of age with a reported first-degree history of probable AD, who were individually matched for their gender, age, and educational level. In comparison with the ε4 noncarriers, the ε4 homozygotes and heterozygotes each had abnormally low CMRgl in the same brain regions as patients with probable AD (Reiman et al. 1996, 2001b). Despite no significant differences in clinical ratings or neuropsychological test scores and no significant interactions between these measurements and time, the ε4 heterozygotes had significantly higher two-year rates of CMRgl decline (Reiman et al. 2001a). Based on these data, we estimated the power of PET to test the efficacy of candidate prevention therapies to attenuate this decline in two years (Reiman et al. 2001a). In complementary PET studies of non-demented ε4 carriers and noncarriers who were about 10 years older, had memory concerns, and had slightly lower MMSE scores, Gary Small and his colleagues found similar baseline abnormalities and longitudinal declines. Furthermore, lower CMRgl measurements in the posterior cingulate and parietal cortex were correlated with a subsequent decline in memory (Small et al. 1995, 2000). While it remains possible that the CMRgl abnormalities reflect aspects of the ε4 allele unrelated to AD, PET studies suggest that these abnormalities are related to the development of this disorder. While there may be a few differences (Mielke et al. 1998; Higuchi et al. 1997), patients with probable AD appear to have a similar pattern of reductions in regional CMRgl whether or not they have the ε4 allele (Corder et al. 1997; Hirono et al. 1998), and, as previously noted, the CMRgl abnormalities in patients with probable AD predicted the subsequent progression of dementia and the histopathological diagnosis of AD (Hoffman et al. 2000; Silverman et al. 2001), were progressive (Jagust et al. 1988; Haxby et al. 1990; McGeer et al. 1990; Smith et al. 1992; Alexander et al. 2002a), and were correlated with dementia severity (Minoshima et al. 1995). Our ongoing longitudinal study promises to clarify the extent to which the CMRgl abnormalities and initial declines in ε4 homozygotes and heterozygotes predict subsequent

Table 1. Number of AD Patients per Treatment Group Needed to Detect an Effect with 80% Power in One Year

	Treatment Effect			
	20%	30%	40%	50%
Frontal	85	38	22	14
Parietal	217	97	55	36
Temporal	266	119	68	44
Cingulate	343	153	87	57
Combined	62	28	16	10

$P=0.01$ (two-tailed) No adjustment for normal aging effects or subject attriton

rates of cognitive decline and conversion to MCI and AD, and it promises to support the use of PET in the efficient evaluation of prevention therapies.

Other promising PET radiotracer techniques have been developed for the study of AD. [^{11}C] methylpiperidinyl propionate (PMP) PET provides estimates of acetylcholinesterase activity and has been used to detect deficits in patients with probable AD. This radiotracer method could be used to evaluate the extent of *central* inhibition by established or investigational acetylcholinesterase inhibitors and help optimize dosage schedules (Kuhl et al. 1999). [^{11}C](R)-PK11195 PET provides estimates of peripheral benzodiazepine receptor binding, a putative marker of neuroinflammation; it has been used to detect abnormally increased measurements and herald the subsequent onset of atrophy in patients with probable AD, and it could be used to track the course of neuroinflammation in AD and characterize the central anti-inflammatory effects of medications (Cagnin et al. 2001). Researchers have recently developed promising PET radiotracer methods for the assessment of AD histopathology (Mathis et al. 2002; Shogi-Jadid et al. 2002; Klunk et al. 2004). Additional research is needed to further evaluate these methods, identify the most suitable radioligands and tracer-kinetic models, and use them to characterize, compare, and track measurements in patients with AD and normal controls.

MRI in the Study of AD

Volumetric MRI studies reveal abnormally high rates of brain atrophy in patients with probable AD, including progressive reductions in the volume of the hippocampus, entorhinal cortex, and whole brain and progressive enlargement of the ventricles and sulci (Seab et al. 1988; Jack et al. 1992, 1997, 1998, 2000; Golomb et al. 1993; de Leon et al. 1989, 1993; Kesslak et al. 1991; Rusinek et al. 1991; Killiany et al. 1993; Lehericy et al. 1994; Deweer et al. 1995; Laakso et al. 1995, 1996; Krasuski et al. 1998; Juottonen et al. 1998, 1999; Schuff et al. 1997; Frisoni et al. 1999; Bobinski et al. 1999; Xu et al. 2000; Visser et al. 1999; Du et al. 2003, 2004; Fox et al. 1996a, 2000, 2001; Freeborough and Fox 1997; Fox and Freeborough 1997). T_1-weighted volumetric MRI measurements of hippocampal, entorhinal cortex, and whole brain volume are currently the most promising and extensively studied structural brain imaging measurements in the early detection and tracking of AD, and they have promising roles in the assessment of candidate treatments to modify disease progression. MRI studies find significantly smaller hippocampal volumes in patients with probable AD (Seab et al. 1988; Jack et al. 1992, 1998; Golomb et al. 1993; de Leon et al. 1989, 1993; Kesslak et al. 1991; Rusinek et al. 1991; Killiany et al. 1993; Lehericy et al. 1994; Deweer et al. 1995; Laakso et al. 1995, 1996; Krasuski et al. 1998; Juottonen et al. 1999; Schuff et al. 1997; Frisoni et al. 1999) and non-demented persons at risk for AD (Kaye et al. 1997; Fox et al. 1996b,c; Convit et al. 1995, 1997; Jack et al. 1999; Du et al. 2001; Soininen et al. 1995; Reiman et al. 1998; Killiany et al. 2000; Schott et al. 2003; Scahill et al. 2002), correlations between reduced hippocampal volume and the severity of cognitive impairment (Kesslak et al. 1991, Keweer et al. 1995; Laakso et al. 1996), and progressive declines in hippocampal volume during the course of the illness (Rusinek et al. 1991; Jack et al. 2000; Du et al. 2001). Methods for the reliable characterization of entorhinal cortex volume have recently been developed and used in the early detection and tracking of MCI and AD (Juottonen et al. 1999; Frisoni et al. 1999; Xu et al. 2000; Du et al. 2001, 2003, 2004). Using these methods, studies have found abnormally small entorhinal cortex volumes in patients with MCI and probable AD. They have also shown that small entorhinal cortex volumes help to predict the rate of conversion to probable AD in patients with MCI (Killiany et al. 2000), that patients with AD have abnormally high annual rates of entorhinal atrophy (Du et al. 2003, 2004) and, depending on how the measurement is made, that the rate of entorhinal cortex atrophy may be greater than the rate of hippocampal atrophy in these patients (Du et al. 2004).

Fox et al. have developed a semi-automated method for the measurement of whole brain atrophy in individual human subjects following the co-registration and digital subtraction (DS) of MRIs (Fox et al. 1996a, 2000; Freeborough and Fox 1997; Fox and Freeborough 1997). They found significantly higher rates of whole brain atrophy in patients with probable AD than those associated with normal aging (Fox et al. 1996a, 2000; Freeborough and Fox 1997; Fox and Freeborough 1997), as well as significantly higher rates of whole brain atrophy shortly before the onset of dementia in persons at risk for AD (Schott et al. 2003; Scahill et al. 2002). They have also estimated the statistical power of this method to test the efficacy of candidate treatments to attenuate these atrophy rates (Fox et al. 2000). We have recently developed and tested a fully automated algorithm for the measurement of brain atrophy from sequential MRIs using an iterative principal component analysis (IPCA) (Chen et al. 2004). We have applied it to the study of patients with AD, our cognitively normal APOE ε4 homozygotes, heterozygotes, and noncarriers, and have begun to apply it to the study of transgenic mice (Chen et al. 2001, 2002a,b; Hauss-Wegrzyniak et al. 2002). Other promising methodological developments for the analysis of volumetric MRIs include, but are not limited to, the use of voxel-based morphometry (VBM) to create probabilistic brain maps to compute regional alterations in gray matter or white matter (Ashburner and Friston 2000; Alexander et al. 2001, 2002b,c), and the use of non-linear warping algorithms to characterize alterations in the size and shape of the hippocampus (Csernansky et al. 2000), multiple brain regions (Fox et al. 2001), variations in gyral and sulcal patterns (Thompson et al. 2001), and reductions in gray matter (Thompson et al. 2001, 2003).

PET and MRI in the Evaluation of Putative AD Treatment

In Temple's commonly cited definition (Temple 1995), "A surrogate endpoint of a clinical trial is a laboratory measurement or a physical sign used as a substitute for a clinically meaningful endpoint that measures directly how a patient feels, functions, or survives. Changes induced by a therapy on a surrogate endpoint are expected to reflect changes in a clinically meaningful endpoint." According to Fleming and DeMets (1996), a valid surrogate endpoint is not just a correlate of the clinical outcome; rather, it should reliably and meaningfully predict the clinical outcome and it should fully capture the effects of the intervention on this outcome. Citing several examples, they note several ways in which an otherwise promising surrogate endpoint might fail to provide an adequate substitute for a clinical endpoint. Although few if any surrogate endpoints have been rigorously validated, the 1997 United States "FDA Modernization Act" authorizes the approval of drugs for the treatment of serious and life-threatening illnesses, including AD, based on its effect on an unvalidated surrogate (US Food and Drug Administration 2002). To promote the study and expedite the approval of drugs for the treatment of these disorders, "fast track approval" may be granted if the drug has an effect on a surrogate marker that is "reasonably likely" to predict a clinical benefit; in this case, the drug sponsor may be required to conduct appropriate post-marketing studies to verify the drug's clinical benefit and validate the surrogate endpoint (US Food and Drug Administration 2002).

FDG PET measurements of posterior cingulate, parietal, temporal, and prefrontal CMRgl and volumetric MRI measurements of hippocampal, entorhinal cortex, and whole brain volume are currently the best-established surrogate markers for the assessment of putative drugs in the treatment of AD. These surrogate endpoints are not rigorously validated, partly because validation may actually require demonstration of these endpoints to account for the predicted clinical effect using several established disease-modifying treatments! Still, these brain imaging measurements are "reasonably likely" to predict a drug's clinical benefit in the treatment of AD. They have much greater statistical power than traditional outcome measures (Alexander et al. 2002a), reducing the potential cost of proof-of-concept studies. They are "reasonably likely" to determine a drug's disease-modifying effects, helping to distinguish a drug's disease-modifying effects from symptomatic effects. As discussed below, these brain-imaging measurements may permit the efficient discovery of prevention therapies in non-demented persons at risk for AD (Reiman et al. 2001a; Fox et al. 2000), and they may assist in the pre-clinical screening of candidate treatments in transgenic mice and other putative animal models of AD (Hauss-Wegrzyniak et al. 2002; Ashburner and Friston 2000). For all of these reasons, FDG PET and volumetric MRI have important and emerging roles in the evaluation of putative disease-modifying candidate drugs in the treatment and prevention of AD.

When using FDG PET in a clinical trial of a putative drug for the treatment or prevention of AD, we recommend the following: 1) the use of a state-of-the-art imaging system with an axial field-of-view that covers the entire brain; 2) data acquisition in the three-dimensional mode, thus permitting the use of lower radiation doses; 3) the use of a non-invasive, image-derived input function, thus permitting the computation of quantitative measurements (in case CMRgl reductions are so extensive that they affect measurements in the whole brain or relatively spared regions, like the pons, that would otherwise be used to normalize images for the variation in absolute measurements); 4) data acquisition in the "resting state" (e.g., eyes closed and directed forward) rather than during the performance of a behavioral task (since the resting state has been used most extensively to track the progression of CMRgl changes in patients with AD and non-demented persons at risk for the disorder and since any effects of a drug on task performance could confound interpretations about the drug's putative disease-modifying effects); 5) the use of an automated brain mapping algorithm to characterize and compare regional CMRgl declines in the active treatment and placebo treatment arms (to date, SPM99 has been the most extensively used algorithm for tracking CMRgl declines in patients with AD and non-demented patients at risk for the disorder); 6) quality assurance procedures to maximize the quality and standardization of image-acquisition and image-analysis procedures at different sites; and 7) a single site for the technical coordination and the centralized storage and analysis of data in multi-center studies.

In the design of clinical imaging trials using FDG PET (and volumetric MRI), we recommend 1) efforts to control or account for potentially confounding effects, such as medication effects (e.g., stratifying samples for use of an approved medication, discouraging the introduction of new medications during the trial, and minimizing or accounting for the use of medications prior to the PET session) and changes in depression ratings; 2) the use of baseline, early, and end-of-treatment scans (performance of the early scan after a drug's steady state and relevant pharmacodynamic effects would help characterize and contrast a medication's state-dependent effects on local neuronal activity or glucose metabolism and its disease-modifying effects); and 3) the use of additional scans as indicated (e.g., to evaluate the time course of an effect, increase statistical power, or incorporate a randomized start or withdrawal design). 4) Although not required, a randomized start or withdrawal design (US food and Drug Administration 2002) could be used to further support a drug's disease-modifying effects. In a randomized start design, patients initially randomized to the placebo arm and treated for an appropriate time are then re-randomized to active medication or placebo; a disease-modifying effect would be inferred if the change in the surrogate endpoint between the beginning and end of the study is significantly smaller in the patients initially randomized to the active treatment arm (i.e., treated longer) than in those subsequently randomized to the active treatment arm. In a randomized withdrawal design, patients initially randomized to the active treatment arm and treated for an appropriate time are then re-randomized to active medication or placebo; a disease-modifying effect would be inferred if the change in the surrogate endpoint is significantly smaller in the patients who were initially randomized to the active treatment arm and subsequently randomized to placebo than in those who were treated with placebo throughout the study. Practically, a randomized start design may be preferred since it may be difficult to justify drug discontinuation in those who believe that the medication has been helpful. 5) Even if the data are not necessary for accelerated drug approval, we strongly recommend efforts to relate a drug's short-term effects on surrogate endpoint (e.g., six-month effects in patients with probable AD or 12-month effects in patients with MCI) to their subsequent clinical course (e.g., subsequent clinical decline in patients with probable AD or three-year conversion rate to probable AD in patients with MCI). This information will help validate the use of these surrogate markers (and support the use of shorter study intervals) for candidate drug and others to be studied in the future. 6) We strongly encourage the combined use of FDG PET and volumetric MRI in the study of a candidate treatment. Using an individual brain imaging technique, there is a small possibility that a drug's effect on a surrogate endpoint might be unrelated to a disease-modifying effect (e.g., an increase in neuronal activity or brain swelling) or that a drug's effect on a surrogate end-point might actually mask its disease-modifying effect (e.g., a contraction in brain size due to a drug's osmotic or perhaps even plaque-clearing effects). The combined used of complementary imaging techniques would provide converging evidence in support of a drug's disease-modifying effects. It would further reduce the small possibility that the drug's effect on an individual surrogate endpoint is unrelated to its effect on disease progression (an advantage in seeking approval for a drug's disease-modifying effect). It would minimize the chance that a drug effect on one of the surrogate endpoints would mask its disease-modifying effects (an advantage in proof-of-concept studies). Embedding both of the these imaging modalities in clinical trials would maximize the chance of validating one or both surrogate endpoints and help support their role in the efficient discovery of primary prevention therapies. We believe that these advantages far outweigh the additional costs and note that both of these imaging modalities are now widely available. 7) Finally, we wish to encourage the application of these imaging techniques to the study of cognitively normal APOE ε4 carriers in primary prevention trials. To conduct primary prevention trials in these subjects, researchers and ethicists may consider two ways to address the risk of providing genetic information to cognitively normal research participants: withholding information from subjects about their genetic risk with their prior informed consent and including persons with *and* without a genetic risk for AD (as we have been done in our naturalistic studies) or counseling potential research subjects about the uncertainties and risks involved in receiving information about their genetic status, obtaining their informed consent to receive this information, and restricting the study to persons at genetic risk for the disorder.

PET in the Study of Cognitively Normal APOE ε4 Carriers and Noncarriers

To study cognitively normal persons at differential genetic risk for AD, we have used newspaper ads to recruit persons who denied any memory concerns and were medically well. The subjects agreed that they would not receive any information about their APOE genotype (since this information cannot be used to predict with certainty whether or when a person will develop AD) and provided their informed consent. Blood samples were then drawn and APOE genotypes characterized. For each APOE ε4 carrier who agreed to participate in our imaging trials, one ε4 noncarrier was matched for his or her gender, age (within three years), and educational level (within two years). The subjects had quantitative FDG PET measurements of CMRgl as they rested quietly with their eyes closed, a volumetric T_1-weighted MRI, a clinical examination, structured psychiatric interview, and depression rating scale, the Folstein Mini-Mental State Examination (MMSE), and batteries of neuropsychological tests and psycholinguistic tasks. In our ongoing longitudinal study, we have begun to acquire these data every two years in 160 cognitively normal, individually matched ε4 homozygotes, heterozygotes, and noncarriers, 47-68 years of age, with a reported first-degree family history of probable AD. In other studies, we have begun to characterize and compare these measurements in cognitively normal ε4 carriers and noncarriers, 20-80 years of age irrespective of their reported family history or probable AD.

Baseline Measurements

We originally sought to test the hypothesis that cognitively normal, late middle-aged APOE ε4 homozygotes, at a particularly high risk of AD, have abnormally low PET measurements in the same brain regions as patients with probable AD (Reiman et al. 1996). APOE genotypes were characterized in cognitively normal persons, 50–65 years of age, with a reported first-degree family history of probable AD. For each of the 11 ε4 homozygotes who agreed to participate in our imaging study, two ε4 noncarriers were matched for their gender, age (within three years), and educational level (within two years). The ε4 homozygotes had a mean age of 55 (range 50–62), a mean MMSE score of 29.4 (range 28–30), and no significant differences from the controls in their clinical ratings or neuropsychological test scores. To characterize regions of the brain with abnormally low CMRgl in patients with probable AD, an automated algorithm was initially used to create a three-dimensional stereotactic surface projection statistical map comparing the data from 37 patients with probable AD and 22 normal controls (mean age 64) provided by researchers at the University of Michigan (Minoshima et al. 1994, 1995). As previously demonstrated, the patients with probable AD had abnormally low CMRgl bilaterally in posterior cingulate, parietal, temporal, and prefrontal cortex, the largest of which was in the posterior cingulate cortex. To characterize regions of the brain with reduced CMRgl in the cognitively normal ε4 homozygotes, the same brain mapping algorithm was used to create a three-dimensional surface projection statistical map comparing the data from our homozygotes and non-carriers; this map was then superimposed onto the map of CMRgl abnormalities in the patients with probable AD (Fig. 1; Reiman et al. 1996). As predicted, the ε4 homozygotes had abnormally low CMRgl bilaterally in the same posterior cingulate, parietal, temporal, and prefrontal regions as the patients with probable AD (Fig. 1; Reiman et al. 1996). The largest reduction was in the posterior cingulate cortex, which is pathologically affected in AD and might provide the earliest metabolic indicator of the predisposition to Alzheimer's dementia (Minoshima et al. 1994). The ε4 homozygotes also had abnormally low CMRgl bilaterally in additional prefrontal regions (Fig. 1), which PET, MRI, and neuropathological studies suggest are preferentially affected during normal aging (Reiman et al. 1996; Kuhl et al. 1982; Salmon et al. 1991; Loessner et al. 1995; Coffey et al. 1992; Terry et al. 1987) and which have led us to postulate that the APOE ε4 allele accelerates normal aging processes that are necessary but not sufficient for the development of AD (Reiman et al. 1996).

We subsequently sought to detect abnormalities in cognitively normal APOE ε4 heterozygotes (Reiman et al. 2001a,b) thus providing a foundation for using PET to efficiently test the potential of candidate primary prevention therapies in this large segment of the population. Eleven cognitively normal ε4 heterozygotes (50-63 years of age, all with the ε3/ε4 genotype) who reported family history of probable AD in a first-degree relative were matched to our original group of ε4 homozygotes and non-carriers for gender, age, and educational level (Reiman et al. 2001b). The ε4 heterozygotes had perfect scores on the MMSE and no impairments in their neuropsychological test scores. Using the same brain-mapping algorithm employed in our original study, the ε4 heterozygotes had significantly reduced CMRgl bilaterally in the same regions of posterior cingulate, parietal, and temporal cortex as patients with probable AD (Fig. 2; Reiman et al. 2001b). Like the ε4 homozygotes, the largest CMRgl reduction was located in the posterior cingulate cortex. Unlike the ε4 homozygotes, the ε4 heterozygotes did not have significant reductions in additional prefrontal regions, which we postulate will be affected at an older age than that observed in the ε4 homozygotes.

We have recently extended these findings to 160 cognitively normal persons in this age group (including 36 ε4 homozygotes, 46 ε4 heterozygotes, and 78 noncarriers) who enrolled in our longitudinal study and are followed every two years (Reiman et al. 2003). As in our earlier reports, the ε4 carriers had abnormally low CMRgl in the posterior cingulate, parietal, temporal, and prefrontal cortex that were not solely attributable to the combined effects of atrophy and partial volume-averaging (Reiman et al. 2003). Lower CMRgl in each of these regions was significantly correlated with ε4 gene dose, which has been related to a higher risk of AD and a lower mean age at the onset of dementia (Reiman et al. 2003).

We have also extended our findings to the comparison of 10 cognitively normal ε4 heterozygotes and 15 ε4 noncarriers, 20-39 years of age, who were recruited irrespective of their reported family history of AD (Reiman et al. 2002a,b). The ε4 heterozygotes had abnormally low CMRgl in the same regions of posterior cingulate, parietal, temporal, and prefrontal cortex, raising new questions about the earliest brain changes involved in the predisposition to AD and new questions about how these early changes are related to the histopathological and physiological brain changes found at older ages (Reiman et al. 2002a). The finding also

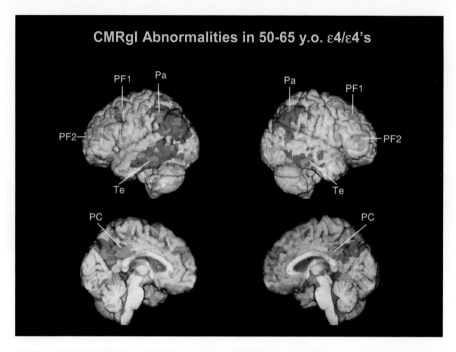

Fig. 1. Regions of the brain with abnormally low CMRgl in late middle-aged, cognitively normal APOE ε4 homozygotes and their relation to brain regions with abnormally low CMRgl in patients with probable AD. In this composite, three-dimensional surface-projection map, purple areas represent abnormally low CMRgl only in the patients with probable AD (relative to their own controls); muted blue areas represent abnormally low CMRgl only in the ε4 homozygotes (relative to their own controls); and bright blue areas reflect abnormally low CMRgl in both the ε4 homozygotes and patients with probable AD. The ε4 homozygotes had abnormally low CMRgl bilaterally in the same regions of posterior cortex (PC), parietal cortex (Pa), temporal cortex (Te), and prefrontal cortex (PF1) as patients with probable AD; they also had abnormally low CMRgl in additional prefrontal regions (PF2), which could reflect accelerated aging. (Adapted with permission from Reiman et al. 1996)

raised the possibility that brain processes associated with the predisposition to AD might be targeted by prevention therapies at a particularly young age and a potentially tractable preclinical stage of disease vulnerability.

We have also begun to characterize and compare MRI measurements in our APOE ε4 carriers and noncarriers. Using volumetric MRIs from the 11 ε4 homozygotes and 22 ε4 non-carriers included in our original analysis of PET data, well-characterized hippocampal landmarks, and a technique used extensively by Mony de Leon and his colleagues at New York University (Fox et al. 2001), we investigated the possibility that cognitively normal persons at risk for AD have reductions in hippocampal volume (Reiman et al. 1998). After normalizing regional measurements for the variation in supratentorial intracranial volume, we found that mean left and right hippocampal volumes were about 8% smaller in the ε4 homozygotes, but did not reach statistical significance. Consistent with other MRI

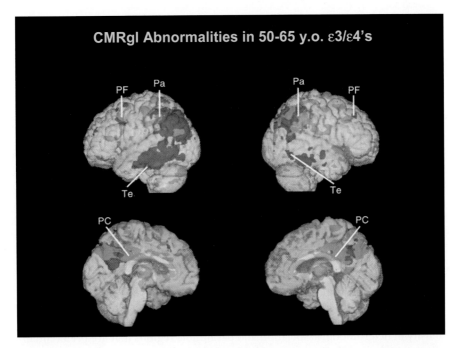

Fig. 2. Regions of the brain with abnormally low CMRgl in cognitively normal, late middle-aged APOE ε4 heterozygotes. The color scheme in this composite, three-dimensional surface-projection map is similar to that described in Figure 1. As indicated in blue, the ε4 heterozygotes (all with the ε3/ε4 genotype) had abnormally low CMRgl bilaterally in the same regions of posterior cortex (PC), parietal cortex (Pa), temporal cortex (Te), and prefrontal cortex (PF) as patients with probable AD.

studies, smaller left and right hippocampal volumes in the 33 subjects were each significantly correlated with lower long-term recall scores. As predicted, posterior cingulate CMRgl measurements continued to distinguish ε4 homozygotes from non-carriers after adjusting for left and right hippocampal volumes in a stepwise logistic regression model. In contrast, neither left nor right hippocampal volumes significantly improved the ability to distinguish the ε4 homozygotes and noncarriers in a model already including posterior cingulate glucose metabolism. Thus, using the image-acquisition and image-analysis techniques employed in this study, PET tended to be more sensitive than MRI in identifying cognitively normal persons at risk for AD. While larger samples and longitudinal assessment are required to confirm our conclusions, we suggest that PET measurements of posterior cingulate CMRgl begin to decline prior to the onset of memory decline in persons at risk for AD, and that MRI measurements of hippocampal volume begin to decline some time later, in conjunction with the onset of memory decline and shortly before the onset of AD (Reiman et al. 1998).

It remains possible that other brain regions, other image-analysis strategies, and longitudinal comparisons could be used to detect abnormalities in MRI measurements of brain volume in cognitively normal persons at genetic risk for AD. We recently used VBM (with procedures optimized to remove the influence of non-brain tissue) to investigate regional abnormalities in gray matter density in the 11 ε4 homozygotes, 11 ε4 heterozytotes, and 22 noncarriers included in our original PET studies. An automated algorithm was used to transform the MRIs into the coordinates of a standard brain atlas, correct the images for non-homogeneities, segment them for gray matter, smoothe them, and create a statistical map of significant differences in gray matter intensity (Alexander et al. 2001). A significance threshold of 0.005, uncorrected for multiple comparisons, was used for hypothesized regional effects. In comparison with the ε4 noncarriers, the ε4 homozygotes had significantly lower gray matter densities in the vicinity of the right posterior cingulate cortex, a right peri-hippocampal region, and the left parahippocampal and lingual gyri. The ε4 heterozygotes had significantly lower gray matter density in the vicinity of the left parahippocampal gyrus, the anterior cingulate cortex, and the right temporal cortex (Alexander et al. 2001). In comparison with the ε4 heterozygotes, the ε4 homozygotes had significantly lower gray matter density in the vicinity of the left parahippocampal and lingual gyri and in bilateral regions of parietal cortex (Alexander et al. 2001). Lower measurements of gray matter density in the left parietal and left parahippocampal/lingual areas were correlated with poorer memory scores in the aggregate ε4 carrier group (Alexander et al. 2001). Thus, cognitively normal ε4 carriers appear to have abnormally low gray matter density in heteromodal association and paralimbic regions that are preferentially affected early in AD. If, as our preliminary findings suggest, reductions in gray matter density are progressive (Alexander et al. 2002b), they could help in the efficient evaluation of primary prevention therapies.

Longitudinal Changes

In our first longitudinal comparison, we characterized and compared two-year CMRgl declines in 10 cognitively normal ε4 heterozygotes and 15 ε4 non-carriers, 50-63 years of age, with a reported first-degree family history of probable AD, and we estimated the power of PET to test the efficacy of treatments to attenuate these declines (Reiman et al. 2001a). There were no significant differences between the subject groups in scores on the MMSE or any of the neuropsychological tests at the time of either scan, no significant declines in these scores between these two times in either group, and no significant Group x Time interactions. The ε4 heterozygotes had significant, two-year CMRgl declines in the vicinity of temporal cortex, posterior cingulate cortex, prefrontal cortex, basal forebrain, parahippocampal/lingual gyri, and thalamus, and these declines were significantly greater than those in the ε4 non-carriers (Reiman et al. 2001a). (Like us, Small and his colleagues found two-year CMRgl declines in their older ε4 carriers with and without a reported family history of probable AD (Small et al. 1995).) Although smaller in magnitude, significant declines in posterior cingulate cortex, parietal cortex, anterior cingulate cortex, and caudate nucleus were found in our group of ε4 noncarriers (Reiman et al. 2001a), apparent physiological markers of normal aging in this age group.

Based on our findings, we have estimated the number of cognitively normal ε4 heterozygotes, 50-63 years of age, per active and placebo treatment group that are needed to detect an attenuation in these CMRgl declines in one or two years (Reiman et al. 2001a; Table 2). As a complement to the power estimates provided in our original report, the tables published here include data for different effect sizes, interpolated estimates of the subjects required in a one-year study, and information about the number of subjects needed to detect an effect in at least one of the implicated regions (denoted in the table as "combined").

In our ongoing longitudinal study, two-year follow-up studies have currently been performed in 94 of our 47 to 68-year-old subjects, including (27 ε4 homozygotes, 27 ε4 heterozygotes, and 40 ε4 noncarriers (Reiman et al. 2003). As in our earlier reports, the ε4 noncarriers had only modest CMRgl declines, and the ε4 carriers had significant CMRgl declines in the vicinity of temporal, posterior cingulate, and prefrontal cortex, basal forebrain, and the thalamus. The CMRgl declines in the temporal and prefrontal cortex in the ε4 carriers were significantly greater than those in the ε4 noncarriers and were significantly correlated with ε4 gene dose. Together, these studies suggest that PET could test the potential efficacy of primary prevention therapies without having to study thousands of research participants, restrict the study to elderly participants, or wait many years to determine whether or when they develop symptoms.

Combining Nick Fox's semi-automated method for the analysis of sequential MRIs, using digital subtraction, and our fully automated method for analysis of sequential MRIs, using IPCA in independent analyses, we have now characterized two-year rates of whole brain atrophy in 36 cognitively normal subjects from our longitudinal study, including 10 ε4 homozygotes, 10 ε4 heterozygotes, and 16 ε4 noncarriers (Chen et al. 2002a). Whole brain atrophy rates were significantly correlated with ε4 gene dose and were significantly greater in the homozygotes than in the noncarriers.

Our ongoing longitudinal PET and MRI study of late middle-aged ε4 homozygotes, heterozygotes, and noncarriers is intended to characterize and contrast the trajectory of decline in brain function and structure in cognitively normal persons at differential risk for AD and to further establish the role of our brain imaging strategy in the efficient evaluation of primary prevention therapies.

Brain Imaging Studies in Transgenic Mice

Transgenic mice containing one or more AD genes develop some of the histopathological features of AD, including amyloid plaques (e.g., Games et al. 1995; Hsiao et al. 1996; Holcomb et al. 1998). Despite their great promise in the study of AD, uncertainties remain about the extent to which transgenic mice provide a model of the disorder or the best way to characterize disease progression. For instance, these mice typically lack some of the histopathological features of AD, amyloid plaques develop relatively early and may not be the strongest correlates of AD severity (Terry et al. 1991; Bierer et al. 1995; Morris et al. 1996), and it is difficult to extrapolate from behavioral observations in laboratory animals to the clinical features of AD.

Table 2. Number of Cognitively Normal APOE-3/4's per Treatment Group Needed to Detect an Effect with 80% Power in Two Years

	Treatment Effect			
	20%	30%	40%	50%
Thalamus	78	35	21	14
Parahippocampal	129	58	33	22
Cingulate	130	58	33	22
Temporal	155	70	40	27
Basal Forebrain	167	75	43	29
Prefrontal	179	80	46	29
Combined	39	19	12	8

P=0.01 (two-tailed), uncorrected for multiple comparisons

We have been interested in the use of functional and structural brain imaging techniques to help bridge the gap between studies of patients with probable AD, cognitively normal persons at risk for AD, and suitable laboratory animals. In transgenic mice, we would like to find neuromaging markers of disease progression that could be used to help screen candidate treatments and further investigate disease mechanisms. Using FDG autoradiography rather than FDG PET (because of its higher spatial resolution), we found that PDAPP transgenic mice overexpressing a mutant form of human APP associated with an autosomal dominant form of AD (Games et al. 1995) had preferentially and progressively reduced activity in the posterior cingulate cortex and relatively spared activity in visual cortex, sensorimotor cortex, cerebellum and brain stem, a pattern observed in patients with probable AD (Reiman et al. 2000; Gonzalez-Lima et al. 2001). Blurring the autoradiographic images to progressively lower resolutions and identifying a non-progressive morphological abnormality (a truncated corpus callosum) in this mouse strain (Valla et al. 2002a), we determined that this abnormality would prevent us from using micro-PET from detecting the posterior cingulate abnormality due to partial-volume effects (Valla et al. 2002a). We have begun to extend this work to a transgenic mouse strain that appears to lack the corpus callosum abnormality (Valla et al. 2002b) in the hope that micro-PET would permit us to track reductions in posterior cingulate activity in the living mouse brain, such that each animal could serve as its own control in the preclinical screening of candidate treatments.

We have also implemented methods for the acquisition of volumetric MRIs in transgenic mice (Chen et al. 2002b; Hauss-Wegrzyniak et al. 2002; Valla et al. 2001). We have adapted our IPCA method to characterize changes in mouse brain volume from sequential MRIs, have demonstrated its ability to detect experimentally reductions in brain volume, and have begun to conduct longitudinal studies in transgenic and wild type mice.

Studies in the Post-Mortem Human Brain

We are also interested in extending findings in patients with AD and cognitively normal persons at genetic risk for AD to studies of the post-mortem human brain. Utilizing cytochrome oxidase histochemistry to investigate metabolic abnormalities in post-mortem brain tissue, our colleagues, Jon Valla and Francisco Gonzalez-Lima, demonstrated that patients with AD have preferential deficits in reductions in cytochrome oxidase activity in every layer of the posterior cingulate cortex (Valla et al. 2001). The largest reduction (36%) was in layer I, which was correlated with dementia severity (Valla et al. 2001). Collaborating with Dietrich Stephan, Joe Rogers, and their colleagues, we have begun to use information from our brain imaging findings to localize brain regions and cells of interest as we investigate genes that are preferentially and differentially expressed in relationship to the histopathological and metabolic features of AD and normal aging, and their interaction with the presence or absence of the APOE ε4 allele. Thus, brain imaging techniques might not only provide an indicator of disease progression that could help in the evaluation of candidate treatments but might also provide new information about the molecular events involved in the pathogenesis of AD and normal aging, including new targets for the discovery of drugs to treat and prevent AD.

Conclusion

In this review article, we have sought to demonstrate how seemingly pedestrian brain imaging markers of disease progression might be used to help in the understanding, early detection and tracking, and treatment and prevention of AD. We are particularly excited about the critical and complementary roles that FDG PET and volumetric MRI could play in the scientific effort to create a world without AD without having to lose a generation along the way.

Acknowledgements

This study was supported by grants from the National Institutes of Health (MH57899-01 and P30 AG19610), the Alzheimer's Association, the Banner Health and Mayo Clinic Foundations, and the Arizona Alzheimer's Research Center.

References

Alexander GE, Chen K, Reiman EM, Caselli RJ, Lewis D, Frost J, Bandy D (2001). Effects of apoli-poprotein E (APOE) e4 on regional brain atrophy in cognitively normal homozygotes (HMZ) and heterozygotes, (HTZ) using voxel-based MRI morphometry. Society for Neuroscience Abstracts 27, 463.9

Alexander GE, Chen K, Pietrini P, Rapoport SI, Reiman EM (2002a) Longitudinal PET evaluation of cerebral metabolic decline in dementia: a potential outcome measure in Alzheimer's disease treatment studies. Am J Psychiat 159:738–745

Alexander GE, Lewis D, Chen K, Reiman EM, Bandy D, Prouty A, Caselli R (2002b) Longitudinal declines of gray matter in cognitively normal apolipoprotein E ε4 homozygotes and heterozygotes evaluated by voxel based MRI Morphometry. Presented at the 8th International Conference on AD and Related Diseases, Stockholm [abstract] Neurobiol Aging 23:S363

American Psychiatric Association (1994) Diagnostic and statistical manual of mental disorders. Fourth edition Washington, DC: American Psychiatric Association

Ashburner J, Friston KJ (2000) Voxel-based morphometry--the methods. Neuroimage 11:805–821.

Bierer LM, Hof PR, Purohit DP, Carlin L, Schmeidler J, Davis KL, Perl DP (1995) Neocortical neurofibrillary tangles correlate with dementia severity in Alzheimer's disease. Arch Neurol 52:81–88

Bobinski M, de Leon MJ, Convit A, De Santi S, Wegiel J, Tarshish CY, Saint Louis LA, Wisniewski HM (1999) MRI of entorhinal cortex in mild Alzheimer's disease. Lancet 353:38–40

Cagnin A, Brooks DJ, Kennedy AM, Gunn RN, Myers R, Turkheimer FE, Jones T, Banati RB (2001) In-vivo measurement of activated microglia in dementia. Lancet 358:461–467

Chen K, Reiman EM, Alexander GE, Crum WR, Fox NC, Rossor MN (2001) Automated method using iterative principle component analysis for detecting brain atrophy rates from sequential MRI in persons with Alzheimer's disease. Soc Neurosci Abstr [abstract]. 27:1261

Chen K, Reiman EM, Domb B, Bandy D, Alexander G, Caselli R, Crum W, Rossor M, Fox N (2002a) Whole brain atrophy rates in cognitively normal persons at genetic risk for Alzheimer's Disease. Presented at the 8th International Conference on AD and Related Diseases, Stockholm [abstract] 23:S349

Chen K, Reiman EM, He T, Alexander G, Galons JP, Stevenson G, Hauss-Wegrzyniak B, Trouard T, Wenk G, Valla J (2002b) Evaluation of an iterative principal component analysis for detecting whole brain volume change in small animal magnetic resonance imaging. Presented at the 8th International Conference on AD and Related Diseases, Stockholm [abstract] Neurobiol Aging 23:S353

Chen K, Reiman E, Alexander G, Bandy D, Renaut R, Fox N, Rossor M. (2004) An automated algorithm for the computation of brain volume change from sequential MRIS using an Iterative Principle Component Analysis and its evaluation for the assesment of whole brain atrophy rates in patients with probable Alzheimer's Disease. Neuroimage, 22 / I pp 134-143

Coffey CE, Wilkinson WE, Parashos IA (1992) Quantitative cerebral anatomy of the aging human brain: a cross-sectional study using magnetic resonance imaging. Neurology 42:527–536.

Cohen D, Eisdorfer C (1988) Depression in family members caring for a relative with Alzheimer's disease. J Am Geriatr Soc 36:885–889

Convit A, de Leon MJ, Tarshish C, De Santi S, Kluger A, Rusinek H, George AE (1995) Hippocampal volume losses in minimally impaired elderly. Lancet 345:266

Convit A, De Leon MJ, Tarshish C, De Santi S, Tsui W, Rusinek H, George A (1997) Specific hippocampal volume reduction in individuals at risk for Alzheimer's disease. Neurobiol Aging 18:131–138

Corder EH, Saunders AM, Strittmatter WJ, Schmechel DE, Gaskell PC, Small GW, Roses AD, Haines JL, Pericak-Vance MA (1993) Gene dose of apolipoprotein E type 4 allele and the risk of Alzheimer's disease in late onset families. Science 261:921–924

Corder EH, Saunders AM, Risch NJ, Strittmatter WJ, Schmechel DE, Gaskell PC Jr, Rimmler JB, Locke PA, Conneally PM, Schmader KE, Small GW, Roses AD, Haines JL, Pericak-Vance MA (1994) Protective effect of apolipoprotein E type 2 allele for late onset Alzheimer disease. Nature Genet 7:180-184

Corder EH, Jelic V, Basun H, Lannfelt L, Valind S, Winblad B, Nordberg A (1997) No difference in cerebral glucose metabolism in patients with Alzheimer disease and differing apolipoprotein E genotypes. Arch Neurol 54:273-277

Csernansky JG, Wang L, Joshi S, Miller JP, Gado M, Kido D, McKeel D, Morris JC, Miller MI (2000) Early DAT is distinguished from aging by high-dimensional mapping of the hippocampus. Dementia of the Alzheimer type. Neurology 55:1636-1643

de Leon MJ, Ferris SH, George AE, Reisberg B, Christman DR, Kricheff II, Wolf AP (1983) Computed tomography and positron emission transaxial evaluations of normal aging and Alzheimer's disease. J Cereb Blood Flow Metab 3:391-394

de Leon MJ, George AE, Stylopoulos LA, Smith G, Miller DC (1989) Early marker for Alzheimer's disease: the atrophic hippocampus. Lancet 672-673

de Leon MJ, Golomb J, George AE, Convit A, Tarshish CY, McRae T, De Santi S, Smith G, Ferris SH, Noz M (1993) The radiologic prediction of Alzheimer's disease: the atrophic hippocampal formation. Am J Neuroradiol 14:897-906

Deweer B, Lehericy S, Pillon B, Baulac M, Chiras J, Marsault C, Agid Y, Dubois B (1995) Memory disorders in probable Alzheimer's disease: the role of hippocampal atrophy as shown with MRI. J Neurol Neurosurg Psychiat 58:590-597

Du AT, Schuff N, Amend D, Laakso MP, Hsu YY, Jagust WJ, Yaffe K, Kramer JH, Reed B, Norman D, Chui HC, Weiner MW (2001) Magnetic resonance imaging of the entorhinal cortex and hippocampus in mild cognitive impairment and Alzheimer's disease. J Neurol Neurosurg Psychiat 71:441-447

Du AT, Schuff N, Zhu XP, Jagust WJ, Miller BL, Reed BR, Kramer JH, Mungas D, Yaffe K, Chui HC, Weiner MW (2003) Atrophy rates of entorhinal cortex in AD and normal aging. Neurology 60:481-486

Du AT, Schuff N, Kramer JH, Ganzer S, Zhu XP, Jagust WJ, Miller BL, Reed BR, Mungas D, Yaffe K, Chui HC, Weiner MW (2004) Higher atrophy rate of entorhinal cortex than hippocampus in Alzheimer's disease. Neurology, 62:422-427

Duara R, Grady C, Haxby J, Sundaram M, Cutler NR, Heston L, Moore A, Schlageter N, Larson S, Rapoport SI (1986) Positron emission tomography in Alzheimer's disease. Neurology 36:879-887

Evans DA, Funkenstein HH, Albert MS, Scherr PA, Cook NR, Chown MJ, Hebert LE, Hennekens CH, Taylor JO (1989) Prevalence of Alzheimer's disease in a community population of older persons: higher than previously reported. JAMA 262: 2551-2556

Farrer LA, Cupples LA, Haines JL, Hyman B, Kukull WA, Mayeux R, Myers RH, Pericak-Vance MA, Risch N, van Duijn CM (1997) Effects of age, sex, and ethnicity on the association between apolipoprotein E genotype and Alzheimer disease. A meta-analysis. APOE and Alzheimer Disease Meta Analysis Consortium. JAMA 278:1349-1356

Fleming TR, DeMets D (1996). Surrogate end points in clinical trials: are we being misled? Ann Intern Med 125:605-613

Foster NL, Chase TN, Fedio P, Patronas NJ, Brooks RA, Di Chiro G (1983) Alzheimer's disease: Focal cortical changes shown by positron emission tomography. Neurology 33:961-965

Fox NC, Freeborough PA (1997) Brain atrophy progression measured from registered serial MRI. J Magn Reson Imaging 7:1069-1075

Fox NC, Freeborough PA, Rossor MN (1996a) Visualization and quantification of rates of atrophy in Alzheimer's disease. Lancet 348:94-97

Fox NC, Warrington EK, Stevens JM, Rossor MN (1996b) Atrophy of the hippocampal formation in early familial Alzheimer's disease. A longitudinal MRI study of at-risk members of a family with an amyloid precursor protein 717Val-Glymutation. Ann NY Acad Sci 777:226-232

Fox NC, Warrington EK, Freeborough PA, Hartikainen P, Kennedy AM, Stevens JM, Rossor MN (1996c) Presymptomatic hippocampal atrophy in Alzheimer's disease: a longitudinal MRI study. Brain 119:2001-2007

Fox NC, Cousens S, Scahill R, Harvey RJ, Rossor MN (2000) Using serial registered brain magnetic resonance imaging to measure disease progression in Alzheimer disease: power calculations and estimates of sample size to detect treatment effects. Arch Neurol 57:333-444

Fox NC, Crum WR, Scahill RI, Stevens JM, Janssen JC, Rossor MN (2001) Imaging of onset and progression of Alzheimer's disease with voxel-compression mapping of serial magnetic resonance images. Lancet 358:201-205

Freebourough PA, Fox NC (1997) The boundary shift integral: an accurate and robust measure of cerebral volume changes from registered repeat MRI. IEEE Trans Med Imaging 16:623-629

Frisoni GB, Laakso MP, Beltramello A, Geroldi C, Bianchetti A, Soininen H, Trabucchi M (1999) Hippocampal and entorhinal cortex atrophy in frontotemporal dementia and Alzheimer's disease. Neurology 52:91-100

Games D, Adams D, Alessandrini R, Barbour R, Berthelette P, Blackwell C, Carr T, Clemens J, Donaldson T, Gillespie F, Guido T, Hagoplan S, Johnson-Wood K, Kahn K, Lee M, Leibowitz P, Lieberburg I, Little S, Masliah E, McConlogue L, Montoya-Zavala M, Mucke L, Paganini L, Penniman E, Power M, Schenk D, Seubert P, Snyder B, Soriano F, Tan H, Vitale J, Wadsworth S, Wolozin B, Zhao J (1995) Alzheimer-type neuropathology in transgenic mice overexpressing V717F β-amyloid precursor protein. Nature 373:523-527

Golomb J, de Leon MJ, Kluger A, George AE, Tarshish C, Ferris SH (1993) Hippocampal atrophy in normal aging - an association with recent memory impairment. Arch Neurol 50:967-973

Gonzalez-Lima F, Berndt JD, Valla J, Games D, Reiman EM (2001) Reduced corpus callosum, fornix and hippocampus in PDAPP transgenic mouse model of Alzheimer's disease. NeuroReport 12:2375-2379

Hauss-Wegrzyniak B, Galons JP, Stevenson G, Wenk G, Chen K, Reiman E, Valla J, Alexander J (2002) Detecting an experimentally induced reduction in mouse brain volume using sequential high-resolution MRI's and the iterative PCA method. Presented at the 8th International Conference on AD and Related Diseases, Stockholm [abstract] Neurobiol Aging 23:S361

Haxby JV, Grady CL, Koss E, Horwitz B, Heston L, Schapiro M, Friedland RP, Rapoport SI (1990) Longitudinal study of cerebral metabolic asymmetries and associated neuropsychological patterns in early dementia of the Alzheimer type. Arch Neurol 47:753-760

Higuchi M, Arai H, Nakagawa T, Higuchi S, Muramatsu T, Matsushita S, Kosaka Y, Itoh M, Sasaki H (1997) Regional cerebral glucose utilization is modulated by the dosage of apolipoprotein E type 4 allele and alpha1-antichymotrypsin type A allele in Alzheimer's disease. Neuroreport 8:2639-2643

Hirono N, Mori E, Yasuda M, Ishii K, Ikejiri Y, Imamura T, Shimomura T, Hashimoto M, Yamashita H, Sasaki M (1998) Lack of association of apolipoprotein E epsilon 4 allele dose with cerebral glucose metabolism in Alzheimer disease. Alzheimer Dis Assoc Disord 12:362-367

Hoffman JM, Welsh-Bohmer KA, Hanson M, Crain B, Hulette C, Earl N, Coleman RE (2000) FDG PET imaging in patients with pathologically verified dementia. J Nucl Med 41:1920-1928

Holcomb L, Gordon MN, McGowan E, Yu X, Benkovic S, Jantzen P, Wright K, Saad I, Mueller R, Morgan D, Sanders S, Zehr C, O'Campo K, Hardy J, Prada CM, Eckman C, Younkin S, Hsiao K, Duff K (1998) Accelerated Alzheimer-type phenotype in transgenic mice carrying both mutant amyloid precursor protein and presenilin 1 transgenes. Nature Med 4:97-100

Hsiao K, Chapman P, Nilsen S, Eckman C, Harigaya Y, Younkin S, Yang F, Cole G (1996) Correlative memory deficits, Aβ elevation, and amyloid plaques in transgenic mice. Science 274:99-102

Jack CR, Petersen RC, O'Brien PC, Tangalos EG (1992) MR-based hippocampal volumetry in the diagnosis of Alzheimer's disease. Neurology 42:183-188

Jack CR Jr, Petersen RC, Xu YC, Waring SC, O'Brien PC, Tangalos EG, Smith GE, Ivnik RJ, Kokmen E (1997) Medial temporal atrophy on MRI in normal aging and very mild Alzheimer's disease. Neurology 49:786-794

Jack CR Jr, Petersen RC, Xu Y, O'Brien PC, Smith GE, Ivnik RJ, Tangalos EG, Kokmen E (1998) Rate of medial temporal lobe atrophy in typical aging and Alzheimer's disease. Neurology 51:993–999

Jack CR Jr, Petersen RC, Xu YC, O'Brien PC, Smith GE, Ivnik RJ, Boeve BF, Waring SC, Tangalos EG, Kokmen E (1999) Prediction of AD with MRI-based hippocampal volume in mild cognitive impairment. Neurology 52:1397–1403

Jack CR Jr, Petersen RC, Xu Y, O'Brien PC, Smith GE, Ivnik RJ, Boeve BF, Tangalos EG, Kokmen E (2000) Rates of hippocampal atrophy correlate with change in clinical status in aging and AD. Neurology 55:484–489

Jagust WJ, Friedland RP, Budinger TF, Koss E, Ober B (1988) Longitudinal studies of regional cerebral metabolism in Alzheimer's disease. Neurology 38:909–912

Juottonen K, Laakso MP, Insausti R, Lehtovirta M, Pitkanen A, Partanen K, Soininen H (1998) Volumes of the entorhinal and perirhinal cortices in Alzheimer's disease. Neurobiol Aging 19:15–22

Juottonen K, Laakso MP, Partanen K, Soininen H (1999) Comparative MR analysis of the entorhinal cortex and hippocampus in diagnosing Alzheimer disease. Am J Neuroradiol 20:139–144

Katzman R, Kawas C (1994) The epidemiology of dementia and Alzheimer disease. In: Terry RD, Katzman R, and Bick KL (eds) Alzheimer disease. New York: Raven Press, pp. 105–122

Kaye JA, Swihart T, Howieson D, Dame A, Moore MM, Karnos T, Camicioli R, Ball M, Oken B, Sexton G (1997) Volume loss of the hippocampus and temporal lobe in the healthy elderly persons destined to develop dementia. Neurology 48:1297–1304

Kesslak J, Nalcioglu O, Cotman C (1991) Quantification of magnetic resonance scans for hippocampal and parahippocampal atrophy in Alzheimer's disease. Neurology 41:51–54

Khachaturian, ZS (1992) The five-five, ten-ten plan for Alzheimer's disease (editorial). Neurobiol Aging 13:197–198

Killiany R, Moss M, Albert M, Tamas S (1993) Temporal lobe regions on magnetic resonance imaging identify patients with early Alzheimer's disease. Arch Neurol 50:949–954

Killiany RJ, Gomez-Isla T, Moss M, Kikinis R, Sandor T, Jolesz F, Tanzi R, Jones K, Hyman BT, Albert MS (2000) Use of structural magnetic resonance imaging to predict who will get Alzheimer's disease. Ann Neurol 47:430–439

Klunk WE, Engler H, Nordberg A, Wang Y, Blomqvist G, Holt DP, Bergström M, Savitcheva I, Huang G-F, Estrada S, Ausén B, Debnath ML, Barletta J, Price JC, Sandell J, Lopresti J, Wall A, Koivisto P, Antoni G, Mathis CA, Långström B (2004) Imaging brain amyloid in Alzheimer's diesease with Pittsburgh Compound-B. Neurology 55:306–319

Krasuski JS, Alexander GE, Horwitz B, Daly EM, Murphy DG, Rapoport SI, Schapiro MB (1998) Volumes of medial temporal lobe structure in patients with Alzheimer's disease and mild cognitive impairment (and in healthy controls). Biol Psychiat 43:60–69

Kuhl DE, Metter EJ, Riege WH, Phelps ME (1982) Effects of human aging on patterns of local cerebral glucose utilization determined by the 18F-fluorodeoxyglucose method. J Cereb Blood Flow Metab 2:163–171

Kuhl DE, Koeppe RA, Minoshima S, Snyder SE, Ficaro EP, Foster NL, Frey KA, Kilbourn MR (1999) In vivo maping of cerebral acetylcholinesterase activity in aging and Alzheimer's disease. Neurology 52:691–699

Laakso MP, Soininen H, Partanen K, Helkala EL, Hartikainen P, Vainio P, Hallikainen M, Hanninen T, Riekkinen PJ Sr. (1995) Volumes of hippocampus, amygdala and frontal lobes in the MRI-based diagnosis of early Alzheimer's disease: correlation with memory functions. J Neural Transm Park Dis Dement Sect 9:73–86

Laakso MP, Partanen K, Riekkinen P, Lehtovirta M, Helkala EL, Hallikainen M, Hanninen T, Vainio P, Soininen H (1996) Hippocampal volumes in Alzheimer's disease, Parkinson's disease with and without dementia, and in vascular dementia: an MRI study. Neurology 46:678–681

Lehericy S, Baulac M, Chiras J, Pierot L, Martin N, Pillon B, Deweer B, Dubois B, Marsault C (1994) Amygdalohippocampal MR volume measurements in the early states of Alzheimer disease. Am J Neuroradiol 15:927–937

Loessner A, Alavi A, Lewandrowski K, Mozley D, Souder E, Gur RE (1995) Regional cerebral function determined by FDG-PET in healthy volunteers: normal patterns and changes with age. J Nucl Med 36:1141–1149

Magistretti PJ, Pellerin L (1996) Cellular bases of brain energy metabolism and their relevance to functional brain imaging: evidence for a prominent role of astrocytes. Cereb Cortex 6:50-61

Mahley RW (1988) Apolipoprotein E: cholesterol transport protein with expanding role in cell biology. Science 240:622–630

Mark RJ, Pang Z, Geddes JW, Uchida K, Mattson MP (1997) Amyloid β-peptide impairs glucose transport in hippocampal and cortical neurons: involvement of membrane lipid peroxidation. J Neurosci 17:1046–1054

Mathis CA, Bacskai BJ, Kajdasz ST, McLellan ME, Frosch MP, Hyman BT, Holt DP, Wang Y, Huang GF, Debnath ML, Klunk WE (2002) A lipophilic thioflavin-T derivative for positron emission tomography (PET) imaging of amyloid in brain. Biorg Med Chem Lett 12:295-298

McGeer EG, Peppard RP, McGeer PL, Tuokko H, Crockett D, Parks R, Akiyama H, Calne DB, Beattie BL, Harrop R (1990)18 Fluorodeoxyglucose positron emission tomography studies in presumed Alzheimer cases, including 13 serial scans. Can J Neurol Sci 17:1-11

McKhann G, Drachman D, Folstein M, Katzman R, Price D, Stadlan EM (1984) Clinical diagnosis of Alzheimer's disease: report of the NINCDS-ADRDA Work Group under the auspices of the Department of Health and Human Services Task Force on Alzheimer's Disease. Neurology 34:939–944

Mega MS, Chen SS, Thompson PM, Woods RP, Karaca TJ, Tiwari A, Vinters HV, Small GW, Toga AW (1997) Mapping histology to metabolism: coregistration of stained whole-brain sections to premortem PET in Alzheimer's disease. Neuroimage 5:147–153

Meguro K, Blaizot X, Kondoh Y, Le Mestric C, Baron JC, Chavoix C (1999) Neocortical and hippocampal glucose hypometabolism following neurotoxic lesions of the entorhinal and perirhinal cortices in the non-human primate as shown by PET. Implications for Alzheimer's disease. Brain 122:1519–1531

Mielke R, Herholz K, Grond M (1994) Clinical deterioration in probable Alzheimer's disease correlates with progressive metabolic impairment of association areas. Dementia 5:36–41

Mielke R, Zerres K, Uhlhaas S, Kessler J, Heiss WD (1998) Apolipoprotein E polymorphism influences the cerebral metabolic pattern in Alzheimer's disease. Neurosci Lett 254:49–52

Minoshima S, Foster NL, Kuhl DE (1994) Posterior cingulate cortex in Alzheimer's disease. Lancet 344:895

Minoshima S, Frey KA, Koeppe RA, Foster NL, Kuhl DE (1995) A diagnostic approach in Alzheimer's disease using three-dimensional stereotactic surface projections of fluorine-18-FDG PET. J Nucl Med 36:1238–1248

Miyata M, Smith JD (1996) Apolipoprotein E allele-specific antioxidant activity and effects on cytotoxicity by oxidative insults and bamyloid peptides. Nature Genet 14:55–61

Morris JC, Storandt M, McKeel DW Jr, Rubin EH, Price JL, Grant EA, Berg L (1996) Cerebral amyloid deposition and diffuse plaques in "normal" aging: Evidence for presymptomatic and very mild Alzheimer's disease. Neurology 46:707–719

Morris JC, Storandt M, Miller JP, McKeel DW, Price JL, Rubin EH, Berg L (2001) Mild cognitive impairment represents early-stage Alzheimer disease. Arch Neurol 58:397–405

Petersen RC, Smith GE, Waring SC, Ivnik, RJ, Tangalos EG, Kokmen E (1999) Mild cognitive impairment: clinical characterization and outcome. Arch Neurol 56:303–308

Piert M, Koeppe RA, Giordani B, Minoshima S, Kuhl DE (1996) Diminished glucose transport and phosphorylation in Alzheimer's disease determined by dynamic FDG-PET. J Nucl Med 37:201–208

Ibanez V, Pietrini P, Alexander GE, Furey ML, Teichberg D, Rajapakse JC, Rapoport SI , Schapiro MB, Horwitz B (1998) Abnormal metabolic patterns in Alzheimer's disease after correction for partial volume effects. Neurology 50:1585–1593

Reiman EM, Caselli RJ (1999) Alzheimer's disease. Maturitas 31:185–200

Reiman EM, Caselli RJ, Yun LS, Chen K, Bandy D, Minoshima S, Thibodeau SN, Osborne D (1996) Preclinical evidence of a genetic risk factor for Alzheimer's disease in apolipoprotein E type 4 homozygotes using positron emission tomography. N Engl J Med 334:752–758

Reiman EM, Uecker A, Caselli RJ, Lewis S, Bandy D, de Leon MJ, De Santi S, Convit A, Osborne D, Weaver A, Thibodeau SN (1998) Hippocampal volumes in cognitively normal persons at genetic risk for Alzheimer's disease. Ann Neurol 44:288–291

Reiman EM, Uecker A, Gonzalez-Lima F, Minear D, Chen K, Callaway NL, Berndt JD, Games D (2000) Tracking Alzheimer's disease in transgenic mice using fluorodeoxyglucose autoradiography. NeuroReport 11:987–991

Reiman EM, Caselli RJ, Chen K, Alexander GE, Bandy D, Frost J (2001a) Declining brain activity in cognitively normal apolipoprotein E ε4 heterozygotes: a foundation for testing Alzheimer's prevention therapies. Proc Natl Acad Sci USA 98:3334–3339

Reiman EM, Caselli RJ, Alexander GE, Chen, K (2001b) Tracking the decline in cerebral glucose metabolism in persons and laboratory animals at genetic risk for Alzheimer's disease. Clin Neurosci Res 1:194–206

Reiman EM, Chen K, Bandy D, Prouty A, Burns C, Alexander G, Caselli R (2002a) Effects of age on cerebral glucose metabolism in APOE E ε4 carriers and noncarriers. Presented at the 8th Internatiomal Conference on AD and Related Diseases, Stockholm [abstract]. Neurobiol Aging 23:S351–S352

Reiman EM, Chen K, Bandy D, Prouty A, Burns C, Alexander G, Caselli R (2002b) Abnormalities in regional brain activity in young adults at genetic risk for late-onset Alzheimer's disease Presented at the 8th International Conference on AD and Related Diseases, Stockholm [abstract]. Neurobiol Aging 23:S421

Reiman EM, Chen K, Alexander GE, Caselli RJ (2003) Positron emission tomography studies of cognitively normal persons at genetic risk for Alzheimer's disease. Presented at the IPSEN Foundation Conference on the Living Brain and Alzheimer's Disease, Paris

Rusinek H, de Leon MJ, George AE, Stylopoulos LA, Chandra R, Smith G, Rand T, Mourino M, Kowalski H (1991) Alzeimer disease: measuring loss of cerebral gray matter with MRI imaging. Radiology 178:109–114

Salmon E, Sadzot B, Maquet P, Dive D, Franck G (1991) Decrease of frontal metabolism demonstrated by positron emission tomography in a population of healthy elderly volunteers. Acta Neurol Belg 91:288-295

Saunders AM, Strittmatter WJ, Schmechel D, George-Hyslop PH, Pericak-Vance MA, Joo SH, Rosi BL, Gusella JF, Crapper-MacLachlan DR, Alberts MJ (1993) Association of apolipoprotein E allele 4 with late-onset familial and sporadic Alzheimer's disease. Neurology 43:1467-1472

Saunders AM, Hulette O, Welsh-Bohmer KA, Schmechel DE, Crain B, Burke JR, Alberts MJ, Strittmatter WJ, Breitner JC, Rosenberg C (1996) Specificity, sensitivity, and predictive value of apolipoprotein-E genotyping for sporadic Alzheimer's disease. Lancet 348:90–93

Scahill RI, Schott JM, Stevens JM, Rossor MN, Fox NC (2002) Mapping the evolution of regional atrophy in Alzheimer's disease: unbiased analysis of fluid-registered serial MRI. Proc Natl Acad Sci USA 99:4703–4707

Schott JM, Fox NC, Frost C, Scahill RI, Janssen JC, Chan D, Jenkins R, Rossor MN (2003) Assessing the onset of structural change in familial Alzheimer's disease. Ann Neurol 53:181-188

Schuff N, Amend D, Ezekiel F, Steinman SK, Tanabe J, Norman D, Jagust W, Kramer JH, Mastrianni JA, Fein G, Weiner MW (1997) Change of hippocampal N-acetyl aspartate and volume in Alzheimer's disease. Neurology 49:1513–1521

Schwartz WJ, Smith CB, Davidsen L, Savaki H, Sokoloff L, Mata M, Fink DJ, Gainer H (1979) Metabolic mapping of functional activity in the hypothalamic neurohypophysial system of the rat. Science 205:723–725

Seshadri S, Beiser A, Selhub J, Jacques PF, Rosenberg IH, D'Agostino RB, Wilson PW, Wolf PA (2002) Plasma homocysteine as a risk factor for dementia and Alzheimer's disease. New Engl J Med 346: 476–483

Seab JP, Jagust WJ, Wong ST, Roos MS, Reed BR, Budinger TF (1988) Quantitative NMR measurements of hippocampal atrophy in Alzheimer's disease. Magn Reson Med; 8:200–208

Shoghi-Jadid K, Small GW, Agdeppa ED, Kepe V, Ercoli LM, Siddarth P, Read S, Satyamurthy N, Petric A, Huang SC, Barrio JR (2002) Localization of neurofibrillary tangles (NFTs) and beta-amyloid placques (APs) in the brains of living patients with Alzheimer's disease. Am J Geriatr Psychiat 10:24–35

Silverman DH, Small GW, Chang CY, Lu CS, Kung De Aburto MA, Chen W, Czernin J, Rapoport SI, Pietrini P, Alexander GE, Schapiro MB, Jagust WJ, Hoffman JM, Welsh-Bohmer KA, Alavi A, Clark CM, Salmon E, de Leon MJ, Mielke R, Cummings JL, Kowell AP, Gambhir SS, Hoh CK, Phelps ME. (2001) Positron emission tomography in evaluation of dementia: Regional brain metabolism and long-term outcome. JAMA 286 :2120–2127

Small GW, Mazziotta JC, Collins MT, Baxter LR, Phelps ME, Mandelkern MA, Kaplan A, La Rue A, Adamson CF, Chang L, et al (1995) Apolipoprotein E type 4 allele and cerebral glucose metabolism in relatives at risk for familial Alzheimer disease. J Am Med Assoc 273:942–947

Small GW, Ercoli LM, Silverman DH, Huang SC, Komo S, Bookheimer SY, Lavretsky H, Miller K, Siddarth P, Rasgon NL, Mazziotta JC, Saxena S, Wu HM, Mega MS, Cummings JL, Saunders AM, Pericak-Vance MA, Roses AD, Barrio JR, Phelps ME (2000) Cerebral metabolic and cognitive decline in persons at genetic risk for Alzheimer's disease. Proc Natl Acad Sci USA 97: 6037–6042

Smith GS, de Leon MJ, George AE, Kluger A, Volkow ND, McRae T, Golomb J, Ferris SH, Reisberg B, Ciaravino J (1992) Topography of crosssectional and longitudinal glucose metabolic defecits in Alzheimer's disease. Pathophysiologic implications. Arch Neurol 49:1142–1150

Snowdon DA, Tully CL, Smith CD, Riley KP, Markesbery WR (2000) Serum folate and the severity of atrophy of the neocortex in Alzheimer disease: findings from the nun study. Am J Clin Nutr 71:993–998

Soininen H, Partanen K, Pitkanen A, Hallikainen M, Hanninen T, Helisalmi S, Mannermaa A, Ryynanen M, Koivisto K, Riekkinen P Sr (1995) Decreased hippocampal volume asymmetry on MRIs in nondemented elderly subjects carrying the apolipoprotein ε4 allele. Neurology 45:391–392

Strittmatter WJ, Weisgraber KH, Huang DY, Dong LM, Salvesen GS, Pericak-Vance M, Schmechel D, Saunders AM, Goldgaber D, Roses AD (1993) Binding of human apolipoprotein E to synthetic amyloid β peptide isoform-specific effects and implications for late-onset Alzheimer disease. Proc Natl Acad Sci USA 90:98–8102

Strittmatter WJ, Weisgraber KH, Goedert M, Saunders AM, Huang D, Corder EH, Dong LM, Jakes R, Alberts MJ, Gilbert JR, Hans S, Hulette C, Einstein G, Schmechel DE, Pericak-Vance MA, Roses AD (1994) Hypothesis: microtubule instability and paired helical filament formation in the Alzheimer disease brain are related to apolipoprotein E genotype. Exp Neurol 125:163–171

Temple R (1995) A regulatory authority's opinion about surrogate endpoints. In: Nimmo WS, Tucker GT (eds) Clinical measurement in drug evaluation. New York, NY, John Wiley & Sons, Ltd, pp. 3–22

Terry RD, DeTeresa R, Hansen LA (1987) Neocortical cell counts in normal human adult aging. Ann Neurol 21:530–539

Terry RD, Masliah E, Salmon DP, Butters N, DeTeresa R, Hill R, Hansen LA, Katzman R (1991) Physical basis of cognitive alterations in Alzheimer's disease: synapse loss is the major correlate of cognitive impairment. Ann Neurol 30:572–580

Terry RD, Maskiah E, Hansen LA(1999) The neuropathology of Alzheimer disease and the structural basis of its cognitive alterations. In: Terry RD, Katzman R, Bick KL, Sisodia SS (eds) Alzheimer disease. Second edition. Philadelphia: Lippincott Williams & Wilkins, pp. 187–206

Thompson PM, Mega MS, Woods RP, Zoumalan CI, Lindshield CJ, Blanton RE, Moussai J, Holmes CJ, Cummings JL, Toga AW (2001) Cortical change in Alzheimer's disease detected with a disease-specific population-based brain atlas. Cereb Cortex 11:1–16

Thompson PM, Hayashi KM, de Zubicaray G, Janke AL, Rose SE, Semple J, Herman D, Hong MS, Dittmer SS, Doddrell DM, Toga AW (2003) Dynamics of gray matter loss in Alzheimer's disease. J Neurosci 23:994–1005

United States Food and Drug Administration. Division of Neuropharmacological Drug Products (2002) Background Document for Joint Advisory Committee Meeting of November 18, 2002: Issues related to the role of brain imaging as an outcome measure in Phase III trials of putative drugs for Alzheimer's Disease.

Valla J, Berndt JD, Gonzalez-Lima F (2001) Energy hypometabolism in posterior cingulate cortex of Alzheimer's patients: superficial laminar cytochrome oxidase associated with disease duration. J Neurosci. 21:4923–4930

Valla J, Chen K, Berndt JD, Gonzalez-Lima F, Cherry SR, Games D, Reiman EM (2002a) Effects of image resolution on autoradiographic measurements of posterior cingulate activity in PDAPP mice: Implications for functional brain imaging studies in transgenic mouse models of Alzheimer's disease. NeuroImage 16:1–6

Valla J, Lewandowski L, Duff K, Reiman EM (2002b) No evidence of significant white matter disruption in the TG2576 mouse model of Alzheimer's disease: implications for *in vivo* microimaging. Presented at the 8th International Conference on AD and Related Disorders, Stockholm, [abstract] Neurobiol Aging 23:S251

Visser PJ, Scheltens P, Verhey FR, Schmand B, Launer LJ, Jolles J, Jonker C (1999) Medial temporal lobe atrophy and memory dysfunction as predictors for dementia in subjects with mild cognitive impairment. J Neurol 246:477–485

Wisniewski T, Castano EM, Golabek A, Vogel T, Frangione B (1994) Acceleration of Alzheimer's fibril formation by apolipoprotein E in vitro. Am J Pathol 145:1030–1035

Xu Y, Jack CR Jr, O'Brien PC, Kokmen E, Smith GE, Ivnik RJ, Boeve BF, Tangalos RG, Petersen RC (2000) Usefulness of MRI measures of entorhinal cortex versus hippocampus in AD. Neurology 54:1760–1767

Subject Index

Printing: Mercedes-Druck, Berlin
Binding: Stein+Lehmann, Berlin